AIDS in French Culture

AIDS in French Culture
Social Ills, Literary Cures

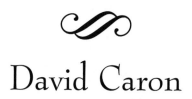

David Caron

The University of Wisconsin Press

The University of Wisconsin Press
1930 Monroe Street
Madison, Wisconsin 53711

www.wisc.edu/wisconsinpress/

3 Henrietta Street
London WC2E 8LU, England

5   4   3   2   1

Printed in the United States of America

Library of Congress Cataloging-in-Publication Data
Caron, David.
      AIDS in French culture : social ills, literary cures /
      David Caron.
      pp.   cm.
      Includes bibliographical references and index.
      ISBN 0-299-17290-2 (cloth: alk. paper)
      ISBN 0-299-17294-5 (paper: alk. paper)
      1. AIDS (Disease)—Social aspects—France.   2. Metaphor.   3. France—Civilization.
   4. AIDS (Disease) in literature.   5. Literature and medicine—France.   6. Homosexuality—
   France.
      I. Title.
      RA643.86.F7 C37   2001
      362.1′969792′00944—dc21   2001001949

For Alex, of course

CONTENTS

ACKNOWLEDGMENTS

It took me a long time to write this book. Naturally, it went through various stages, and at every step of the way I was lucky to find teachers, colleagues, and friends who were amazingly helpful and supportive. First I want to thank David Carroll and Leslie Rabine, who read the manuscript in its earliest stages and convinced me that it was good and that it was worth it. Then came my colleagues at the University of Michigan. Jarrod Hayes, Juli Highfill, Marie-Hélène Huet, Bill Paulson, Frieda Ekotto, Carina Yervasi, and Alain Martinossi have my undying gratitude for their support and friendship. I am well aware of how fortunate I am to have had such extraordinary colleagues. Thank you all for blurring the boundary between work and friendship. I also want to thank Mireille Rosello and James Creech for their helpful reading and precious advice in the final stages of the manuscript, as well as Raphael Kadushin and the staff at the University of Wisconsin Press. Naturally, I am forever indebted to my family for their constant support. Very special thanks also go to Annabelle Cocollos for her talent (next time!) and friendship, and to Thierry Péryoitte and Anna Sciuto without whom Paris would have long ceased to be the city of love. And there is Ross Chambers. What can I possibly say? Thanks for everything.

This book is also dedicated to all those who have suffered from AIDS one way or another.

Parts of this book have previously been published as articles. Segments of chapter 5 appeared as "Playing Doctors: Refiguring the Doctor-Patient Relationship in Hervé Guibert's AIDS Novels," *Literature and Medicine* 14, no. 2 (fall 1995): 237–49, © 1995 The Johns Hopkins University Press. Most of the conclusion appeared as "Liberté, Egalité, Séropositivité: AIDS, the French Republic and the Question of Community," *French Cultural Studies* 9, no. 3 (Oct. 1998): 281–93, © 1998 Alpha Academic.

AIDS in French Culture

Introduction

Where Does AIDS Come from?

The epidemic of metaphors triggered in July 1981 by the first public reports of what would turn out to be the AIDS epidemic spread with far greater speed and efficiency than the virus itself. While we are repeatedly told that sorting facts from fictions is the simplest way to fight AIDS, we are simultaneously reminded that to do so is not simple at all. The combination of a virus and the collapse of the immune system was quick to be conceptualized with tropes of war and nationalism, of spying and counterspying. Because a horrible and untimely death was long thought to be the inevitable outcome of the syndrome, AIDS was also depicted with tropes borrowed from popular literary and film genres, such as detective stories, horror, melodrama, and science fiction, all of which provided reassuring narratives of good and evil wherein evil is eventually vanquished and order restored.[1] Moreover, because it was originally associated with cultural others, such as sexual and ethnic minorities, as well as drug users and foreigners, AIDS incorporated the metaphorical networks and narrative structures already in place in Western cultures to depict, define, and make sense of homosexuality, blackness, addiction, Africa, and, as the epidemic progressed, femaleness. Concurrently with the use of cultural tropes to make sense of the medical event that is the AIDS epidemic, AIDS itself was used as a metaphor in order to make sense of the various cultural, social, and national contexts in which it emerged. AIDS, then, could be a metaphor for the collapse of moral values in modern societies, or for the Cold War, or for the dangers of the excessive social and geographical mobility of populations in today's globalized world.[2] Metaphors, in short, have permeated all sorts of discourses about AIDS. One would be hard-pressed to find a single discourse, whether popular or scientific, literary or technical, oppressive or resistant, that has been able to engage HIV and AIDS without the use of metaphors.

Where did these metaphors come from? What is their relation to the symbolic and social structures from which they emerged? To what extent does modern medical discourse, as it has been elaborated since the second half of the nineteenth century, frame and determine our current experience of AIDS beyond its medical dimension? And what is the cultural specificity of France within that general experience? Or, to put it in blunt terms: Why is it that France has been, by far, the European nation with the highest rate of HIV and AIDS? What is the link between medical discourse, on the one hand, and the production of communities, national or otherwise, on the other? What role did (and does) medical discourse play in defining such communities and in deciding who shall belong to them and who shall not? What is the role of literature, and specifically of the novel, in that enterprise? If, in the late nineteenth century, the French novel was entrusted with the mission of naturalizing bourgeois power in France, can it also be used to propose a counterdiscourse from the margins of that power? In other words, can the novel contribute to the fight against AIDS and, if so, how? This book is an attempt to answer these questions by studying the intersections of three discourses, the literary, the medical, and the political, and by tracing the origin of French AIDS discourses in Third Republic anxieties about nationhood, masculinity, and sexuality. More specifically, I contend that the late-nineteenth-century construction of male homosexuality provided the conceptual and rhetorical frameworks within which AIDS discourses and counterdiscourses were produced and disseminated in contemporary French culture.

Metaphors of Science

From the end of the eighteenth century, the practice, the purpose, and the language of medicine began to change along with other areas of Western cultures. No longer considered an art, medicine progressively acquired the status of science and entered a process of rapid progress and revolutionary discoveries. Strengthened by its newfound prestige, medical discourse began to occupy a central part in overall bourgeois discourse. In postrevolutionary France, following the decentralization and rejuvenation of what was now becoming a profession, doctors began to enjoy an increasingly important social position. With the advent of the Third Republic, doctors made up the second largest professional background of politicians, after lawyers.[3] Nineteenth-century doctors, it seems, were concerned with a lot more than just healing their patients: they were, directly and indirectly, involved in the production and enforcement of cultural and ideological metaphors.

Bourgeois power soon identified, in scientific discourse in general and in biomedical discourse in particular, the possibility of legitimating itself and ensuring its own survival. The *ancien régime,* just overthrown by the French bourgeoisie, had found its justification in religion and the notion of divine right, as theological discourse provided the master discourse and the transcendent authority to interpret nature and the world globally. The new regime now turned to the naturalizing power of science to seek its own justification within a new global explanation of nature, one based on reason, empirical sciences, and demonstrable truth. Just like theological discourse in pre- and early modern times, it soon became the ultimate reference which all sorts of other disciplines and discourses might use to authenticate themselves: philosophical and social theories, the arts, the law, politics, and even literary criticism—all these and more began to gauge their own validity by how well they incorporated and mimicked the methods and language of science. There was no consensus, however, and we know that science didn't replace religion altogether. In fact, both discourses are still cohabitating today, albeit uneasily. Yet, whether in direct competition with theological discourse or in collusion with it, biomedical discourse provided, by and large, the ultimate validation of late-nineteenth-century bourgeois power.

This supreme influence is largely due to the fact that biomedical discourse was perceived as being uncontaminated by subjectivity or any other kind of cultural interference or noise. Unmarked, perfectly objective, it was considered, in a sense, as close to pure reality as language can possibly get. This is what was understood as scientific discourse at the time, and this is the status that modern medicine had acquired. By and large, the ideal of a pure objectivity of scientific discourse remained unquestioned roughly until the end of World War II, when the "discovery" of the Holocaust and the progressive collapse of colonial empires seriously challenged the hegemony of Western thought and its claims to universality. Today, science has been increasingly subjected to radical critiques, often coming from just those social categories that had been defined as subaltern and marginalized by scientific discourses: women, homosexuals, racial and colonial others, and so on. Many now believe that these scientific discourses have been shaped in part by external demands and are in fact always subjective and contaminated by metaphoricity.

In his landmark study, *The Structure of Scientific Revolutions,* published in 1962, Thomas Kuhn proposed a new explanation of scientific progress. Traditionally conceived as a linear and teleological movement that takes us, one discovery after another, closer and closer to complete knowledge of the world, scientific progress, Kuhn argues, is really the result of paradigm shifts. In the Kuhnian sense, a paradigm is a worldview that prevails in a given historical context and mediates our experience of reality; the state of science is a reflection of that worldview and not of the distance separating us from complete and absolute knowledge of the truth. A paradigm, then, predetermines the field of scientific knowledge as well as the empirical gaze of the scientist. According to Kuhn, "What a man sees depends both upon what he looks at and also upon what his previous visual-conceptual experience has taught him to see" (113). From a discursive standpoint, and insofar as a paradigm always predates the gaze, it is therefore impossible for science to propose a purely descriptive type of language that would be able to render an empirically observed reality. For Kuhn: "No language thus restricted to reporting a world fully known in advance can produce mere neutral and objective reports on 'the given.' Philosophical investigation has not yet provided even a hint of what a language able to do that would be like" (127).

More recently, Donna Haraway described the structural role of metaphors in the elaboration of paradigms. She writes: "A metaphor is the vital spirit of a paradigm (or perhaps its basic organizing relation)."[4] In other words, a metaphor gives a system its coherence by concentrating it entirely within a single image. For example, society is a machine or a house or a body—and vice versa.[5] The argument, which I shall not attempt to demonstrate again but, rather, take as my theoretical starting point, is that without a central, structural metaphor there is no system at all: the metaphor performs the system into existence; it doesn't merely express it.[6]

Along a line of thought similar to that of Kuhn and Haraway, Evelyn Fox Keller proposes a critique of what she calls the "science-gender system." In *Reflections on Gender and Science,* she shows how scientific discourse metaphorically represents (and enforces) the values of the system from which it emerged: "Scientists, as human actors, find some pictures or theories more persuasive and even more self-evident than others in part because of the conformation of those pictures or theories to their prior emotional commitments, expectations, and desires" (10). For Kuhn, Haraway, Keller, and others, scientific discourse is, in effect, both a product of and a metaphor for a given worldview organizing a given society at a given historical time. In what relative proportions does this discourse reflect, incorporate, enforce, and/or perform the social order? That, of course, remains to be determined. But one can be sure of one thing: science always tells us something about the fundamental principles and cultural values structuring society.

In the specific context of late-nineteenth-century French society, several structural metaphors come to mind, beyond the more traditional and enduring body metaphor. To compare society to a machine emphasizes social cohesion and efficiency based on a strict distribution of social roles. To think of society as a house, in the sense of both home and building, stresses moral values and harmony in what could be a patriarchal, family-like organization. It is easy to see why both "machine" and "house" provided meaningful metaphors in the historical context of the industrial revolution and bourgeois domesticity, and why they were particularly effective in performing a new social order. Eventually, these metaphors combined into a paradigmatic relation in which the nation, the body, the machine, and the house could all be metaphors for each other, and bourgeois society could achieve a certain degree of systemic cohesion.

No metaphor, however, has had as much naturalizing power as the body metaphor, simply because the body, like nature, is always conceived as ahistorical by definition. But it, too, has gone through a historical process of transformations, and modernity has assigned new metaphorical functions to the human body. In *Making Sex,* Thomas Laqueur explains how the notion of sex changed radically in modern times. According to Laqueur, until the end of the eighteenth century, women were viewed in terms of sameness, according to what he calls the one-sex model. Anatomically, the female sex was seen as only an imperfect, inverted version of the male sex. Gender, not sex, was then the significant marker of radical difference with which male domination over women was enforced; or as Laqueur writes: "Sex . . . was still a sociological and not an ontological category" (8). After the eighteenth century, women came to be conceived in terms of difference, according to a two-sex model in which each sex became an autonomous ontological entity with its own physiological and moral characteristics. But beyond the issues of sex and gender, this paradigm shift suggests that a radical change has occurred in Western conceptualizations of the human body as a whole.

In the field of medicine, the progressive disappearance of the older paradigm of the human body pushed the immanent concepts of health and disease away from center stage as attention focused on bacteriological and virological research, that is, on fields structured by notions of sameness and difference, inside and outside. As Michel Foucault points out in *Birth of the Clinic,* "new" diseases even began to appear at the time. What characterizes this new paradigm is that it assigned an ontological value to the human body. Logically, biology and medicine found themselves invested with a social role they had not heretofore possessed. As Laqueur points out: "Biology—the stable, ahistorical sexed body—is understood to be the epistemic foundation for prescriptive claims about the social order" (6). And according to Foucault:

> Generally speaking, it might be said that up to the end of the eighteenth century medicine related much more to health than to normality. . . . Nineteenth-century medicine, on the other hand, was regulated more in accordance with normality than with health . . . and physiological knowledge, once marginal and purely theoretical knowledge for the doctor— was to become established (Claude Bernard bears witness to this) at the very center of all medical reflexion. . . . one did not think first of the internal structure of *the organized being,* but of *the normal and the pathological.* (35; original emphasis)

To the extent that the body was where social order was to be articulated in terms of sameness and difference, the health/disease dichotomy automatically signified much more than the momentary condition of a given body: it came to represent and distribute the natural characteristics of the Same and the Other. The medical gaze, then, became subject to an equally radical transformation. As I will discuss in greater detail throughout the coming chapters, one of the missions of nineteenth-century medicine was to identify the physical marks of otherness on the bodies of "perverts," "degenerates," "Jews," and so on, thus creating the categories it claimed merely to observe and describe. Medical rhetoric, therefore, is also performative, and the body becomes the metaphorical site of social and political projects.

Both terms of the metaphor, however, are affected (or infected) by their coming into contact with one another. As Haraway remarks: "Analogy and primary referent are both altered in meaning as a result of juxtaposition" (10); and Mary Hesse gives the following example: "Nature becomes more like a machine in the mechanical philosophy, and actual concrete machines are seen as if stripped down to their essential qualities of mass in motion."[7] If we examine the metaphor of the bourgeois nation-state as body, we can observe a similar kind of mutual contamination of the terms. The body-as-bourgeois-nation becomes ideally balanced, moderate, private, and civilized. The bourgeois-nation-as-body has natural boundaries; it consumes, expels waste, seeks normality, reinforces its defenses, fights foreign bodies, and fully realizes itself in the process of reproduction. Thanks to their metaphorical contact, body and nation can exchange their respective qualities: the body is now the object of social control and domestication, while the nation can go wild, as it were, and claim the necessity to satisfy its instinctive and natural needs in order to ensure its health and survival. In the specific context of late-nineteenth-century France, for example, this metaphor may translate into applying the concept of degeneracy to internal politics in order to exert social control, or summoning the principles of evolution to justify imperialist expansion and colonization. The metaphor, then, is complemented by a synecdoche allowing the empirical descriptions of individual clinical cases to make sense within discourses and disciplines concerned with the collective. In other words, the individual is a representative of the species. Such rhetorical displacement is, in fact, the condition for the emergence of discourses on homosexuality and Jewishness (discussed in later chapters) in the second half of the nineteenth century.

The AIDS crisis has at the same time brought on a crisis of that whole rhetorical apparatus of knowledge and power. We know that in classical rhetoric, the purpose of a metaphor is to clarify an excessively complex idea by lending it a simpler, more familiar form. The frequent use of analogies to explain difficult scientific notions is a good example of that. Think, for instance, of the many ways the actions of HIV on the immune system have been explained to us in the media. But with AIDS science, the complex original to be simplified for comprehension's sake was never really there in the first place; or at least it was seriously in doubt and did not constitute an uncontested body of knowledge, fully mastered by experts and ready to be transmitted down to us, laypersons, via simple figures, images, and storylines. In fact, metaphors and other tropes began to occupy the vulnerable and half-empty space of the original—to infect it, as it were. Because of this blurring of categories and the increasing difficulty we have in distinguishing an original scientific fact (the knowledge of which determines power) and its metaphorical rendition (destined for the unknowing masses and therefore linked to their subjugation), the AIDS crisis has allowed a radical critique of the way disease metaphors have been used to establish and enforce power. In a sense, many AIDS counterdiscourses have, in effect, turned metaphors back against the system that produced them, thus exposing the role of medical science in naturalizing bourgeois power and marginalized identities.

Two Models of Health and Disease

Although the transformation of medicine into a scientific discipline is concomitant with modernity and the bourgeoisie's rise to political power, medical thought in the nineteenth century was still inscribed within the frames of two ancient notions, as described by Georges Canguilhem.[8] One was elaborated in ancient Egypt and posits the body as inherently healthy until the intrusion or loss of a localizable element causes the illness. This ontological entity must then be located, and either expelled or restored. As Canguilhem writes: "Disease enters and leaves man as through a door" (39) ["La maladie entre et sort de l'homme comme par la porte" (11)]. The other concept, of Greek origin, defines both illness and health as a matter of internal dynamics and balance. From that conceptual standpoint, disease is not an ontological other, and to restore the patient's health one needs to rectify the internal imbalance that caused the illness. In this model, Canguilhem adds,

> disease is not simply disequilibrium or discordance; it is, and perhaps more importantly, an effort on the part of nature to effect a new equilibrium in man. Disease is a generalized reaction designed to bring about a cure; the organism develops a disease in order to get well. (40–41)

> [La maladie n'est pas seulement déséquilibre ou dysharmonie, elle est aussi, et peut-être surtout, effort de la nature en l'homme pour obtenir un nouvel équilibre. La maladie est réaction généralisée à intention de guérison. (12)]

From these two ancient notions of health and disease, two different conceptions of medicine developed that are still largely operative today. Totalizing medicine, on the one hand, is based on the Greek model of internal dynamics, while localizationist medicine is based on the Egyptian ontological model. Immunology, for example, corresponds to the first model, whereas virology belongs to the second. Yet, for Canguilhem,

> these two conceptions do have one point in common: in disease, or better, in the experience of being sick, both envision a polemical situation: either a battle between the organism and a foreign entity, or an internal struggle between opposing forces. (41; translation modified)

> [Ces deux conceptions ont pourtant un point commun: dans la maladie, ou mieux dans l'expérience de l'être malade, elles voient une situation

polémique, soit une lutte de l'organisme et d'un être étranger, soit une lutte intérieure de forces affrontées. (13)]

While the ontological model became particularly important thanks to the numerous discoveries of external pathogenic agents in the nineteenth century, this does not mean that the dynamic model has fallen into obsolescence. Rather, modern medical disciplines have claimed their respective fields along the same ancient division. Interestingly, AIDS has functioned in both categories, because it was initially conceptualized within the field of immunology before the discovery of HIV made AIDS research fall mostly into the domain of virology.

As AIDS critic Cindy Patton points out in *Inventing AIDS,* these two medical models have generated two different sets of cultural and political tropes, and one of them may dominate at a given historical time. Take the period from the mid-1940s through the 1950s in the United States, for example. The fight against polio, the fear of communist infiltration, and the popularity of Martians in movies and elsewhere were all structured by the same narrative framework, in which all perils were supposed to come from outside and take the form of radical otherness. Evil was another being with whom we were in competition. Now take the 1960s and early 1970s. Immunology, Patton remarks, became more prominent at the time, and so did holistic medicine. These were the years of the Civil Rights movement and student rebellions, of the war on poverty, of global ecological concerns, and so forth. Popular culture, such as Hollywood movies, turned its attention away from outer space and tended to focus inward on political paranoia and conspiracies in which our own government was usually the bad guy. In other words, the source of social problems was now located within society itself. Evil was no longer an ontological other but an immanent aspect of ourselves. To be sure, evil and disease were still clearly considered undesirable, and therefore some kind of Other, but the status of their otherness seemed somewhat different.

For Canguilhem, localizationist medicine reflects "the persistence of a reaction to disease [*mal*] as old as man himself" (40) ["la persistance d'une réaction devant le mal aussi vieille que l'homme lui-même" (12)], which is a desire to localize and define in order to act:

> Without wishing to detract from the grandeur of Pasteur's tenets, we can say without hesitation that the germ theory of contagious disease has certainly owed much of its success to the fact that it embodies an ontological representation of sickness. After all, a germ can be seen, even if it requires the complicated mediation of a microscope, stains and cultures, while we would never be able to see a miasma or an influence. To see an entity is already to foresee an action. (39–40)

[Sans vouloir attenter à la majesté des dogmes pasteuriens, on peut bien dire que la théorie microbienne des maladies contagieuses a dû certainement une part non négligeable de son succès à ce qu'elle contient de représentation ontologique du mal. Le microbe, même s'il lui faut le truchement compliqué du microscope, des colorants et des cultures, on peut le voir, au lieu qu'on ne saurait voir un miasme ou une influence. Voir un être c'est déjà prévoir un acte. (12)]

The semantic duality of the French word *mal,* both "evil" and "disease," should, I think, be restored here, as it emphasizes the metaphorical dimension of such medical concepts; as for the word *être* ("entity"), it clarifies the ontological definition of otherness at work in this case. In short, we are dealing in the same breath with a triple perception of disease, evil, and otherness framed by the dichotomies of inside and outside, and presence and absence. This perception, it seems, must be different when it comes to totalizing medicine. According to Patton, for example: "Immunology was not so much about the Other as about the marginally different that had already been admitted to close proximity" (*Inventing AIDS,* 60). But how different are these two types of Other? On the one hand, it is undeniable that the Other is always produced by the Same, often through a simple and fairly legible process of antithesis, and therefore tells us more about the Same than it does about the Other. In fact, if the Other were truly so, that is, not produced by our symbolic system, one would be unable to conceptualize it or say anything directly about it. On the other hand, the type of otherness produced by a totalizing narrative framework like that of immunology seems to recognize that otherness is in fact performed by purely internal dynamics. Does that mean that such a narrative model simultaneously produces its own, self-critical discourse? What, then, does it tell us about the idea of sameness that is performed in the same gesture? Does the virological, or ontological, narrative, structured by the inside/outside dichotomy, perform the same sameness, so to speak, as the immunological, or dynamic, model?

For Cindy Patton, "[a]lthough science operates as if these two ways of medical thinking are compatible, each in fact carries incompatible cultural meanings and political metaphors" (*Inventing AIDS,* 58). While Patton doesn't imply that one model may be politically and morally more desirable than the other, one can still wonder whether it is possible to use these two metaphorical networks without changing one's ideological position. Indeed, in political terms, the articulation may not be as clear-cut as my earlier examples suggested. It is true that, metaphorically, virology can justify ideological tenets usually associated with the political Right, such as xenophobia, racism, anti-Semitism, and punitive immigration laws, but it may also be reclaimed subversively to undermine hegemonic power structures by infecting them. It is true also that the immunological model can provide the narrative support for progressive politics of social reform and justice, usually thought to belong to the Left's set of values. Yet it can also be used to justify the return to a strict moral order and to issue calls for increased social control, this time in the name of religion.

Consider the example of what is usually called "sexual orientation." The dreary debates around the causes of sexual orientation articulate themselves within the same binary structure: either the internal dynamic of choice or the radical ontology implied by innateness. Both explanations are politically and morally neutral in themselves, and both may be used either homophobically or to improve the social status of gays and lesbians. The political value of each explanatory model resides entirely in its usage. If today one model may be used predominantly by the Right and the other by the Left, it was not and will not always be the case. AIDS, once again, is an interesting example of such rhetorical and political ambivalence. In right-wing discourses the epidemic is said to have occurred either because the modern world has turned away from its traditional set of basic moral values (that is, conceptualized according to the immunological model), or as a result of lax immigration policies (following the virological model). In France, the AIDS discourse of Jean-Marie Le Pen's Front National, for instance, has oscillated between the two rhetorical models according to its strategic concerns and electoral designs.

French Novels and the Construction of Otherness

This book begins with the early decades of the Third Republic, when the literary and political uses of health and disease tropes reached a frenzied peak in French culture. In the years following the humiliating defeat of the Second Empire in the Franco-Prussian War of 1870 and culminating with the Dreyfus affair, France was going through a period of intense national identity crisis. At the same time, capitalism was experiencing its first major crises. The newly created Republic was unstable, and the regime was still fiercely contested by various (and often incompatible) forces bent on overthrowing the republican regime altogether. The rhetorical models provided by the two conceptions of health and disease helped frame opposing views of the ideal national community, one based on the notion of shared social values, the other on an ontological type of organic national identity. In those years, ideological camps were defining and organizing themselves, and preparing the ground for the great confrontations of the twentieth century. Literary and medical discourses were on the frontlines of these ideological battles, as they attempted to diagnose the nature of the social ills affecting French society and to propose solutions. At stake was nothing less than the ultimate definition of Frenchness and nationhood for the future.

I have chosen for analysis, in addition to medical and critical texts, an emblematic novel from that defining period in modern French cultural history: Emile Zola's *La débâcle* (1892), a literary work that epitomizes the dynamic logic of the republican ideal of the French Revolution as well as the normalizing sexual politics entrenched in it. Squarely situating himself against the new brand of nationalism spearheaded by Maurice Barrès and the like, Zola refused to blame social ills on a radical cultural Other, namely the Jews. Instead, he located the source of, and solution to, France's problems within the national community itself. *La débâcle,* a controversial account of the French defeat in 1870 and the penultimate volume in his Rougon-Macquart saga, was Zola's most successful book up to that time and remained his best-selling novel for decades. More than any of Zola's other works of fiction, the text presents itself as a cure, premised on the accuracy of its diagnosis, to whatever ails the nation, and it attempts to authenticate its performative power thanks to medical discourse. In other words, it uses tropes of health and disease to structure its own textuality as well as to envision (and perform) a renewed and "healthy" national community. With the metaphor of degeneration and the figure of the "homosexual," Zola sees the disease of the body politic as internally produced. Cultural fears, it seems, are inextricably linked to gender indecision and anxiety about masculinity, the phenomenon we now identify as "queer." For Zola, unlike the anti-Semites he so vocally opposed at the time of the Dreyfus affair, otherness was a threat that loomed not across national or cultural boundaries but within the nation itself as its co-constitutive darker side. Zola's queer Other, then, is less an ontological entity than a dynamic process of becoming. Yet, while its ideology is undoubtedly exclusionary, Zola's text is eventually undermined by the instability of its rhetorical model, as it unwittingly ends up repositioning in a positive way what it had identified as the very cause of all social ills, degeneration itself.

About one hundred years later, dominant discourses on AIDS in France have drawn extensively from that discursive model. In many countries and cultures, the viral conceptualization of AIDS following the discovery of HIV has generated metaphors that placed the blame for the epidemic on a wide array of extrinsic Others metonymically assimilated to the virus itself. France did not escape that trend, of course, and tropes of viral invasion began to appear from various corners of society, most notably (although not only) from the growing ranks of anti-immigration, extreme-right sympathizers. Yet the intrinsic or immunological conceptualization never really disappeared and has in fact continued to provide a metaphorical framework for AIDS discourses in France.

Several historical and political reasons may explain this peculiarity. For one thing, as the centennial celebration of the publication of "J'accuse" has made clear, Zola still embodies the core value of the French republic—universal integration. The Front National contradicted this republican ideal when it appropriated contamination metaphors to justify its exclusionary politics; thus, these tropes were unacceptable within mainstream public discourses. Finally, and more important, because from its onset the AIDS epidemic has been largely associated with sex between men, it has been framed in a way that draws on early Third Republic constructions of male homosexuality itself, that is, as something that, in modern France, does not constitute a stable ontological category. While blaming Zola for the AIDS epidemic would be a slight overstatement, it does appear, however, that the rhetorical and ideological frameworks of AIDS discourses in France were in fact laid out about a hundred years before, and that the study of Third Republic culture around the time of the Dreyfus affair can tell us a great deal about the way contemporary France has dealt with the epidemic.

In subsequent chapters, I explore what happens when one writes from the point of view of the degenerate—when the governing principle behind a novel is no longer to normalize but to destabilize, no longer to heal society but to infect it. Jean Genet's *Journal du voleur* and Hervé Guibert's *A l'ami qui ne m'a pas sauvé la vie* and *Le protocole compassionnel* challenge not only the different notions of community represented by Third Republic culture, but also, and more important, what neither Zola nor his opponents would have disputed. Indeed, while early Third Republic authors often differed on how to define health and disease, they did agree on the basic premises that the nation was indeed sick, that it should be restored to health, or normality, and that this should be done by absorbing the normalizing power of medical discourse into literature. However, as they flauntingly embody pathological constructions of male homosexuality and strategically reiterate these structuring metaphors, Genet and Guibert subvert them, and expose the exclusionary nature of modern representations of disease as well as the mechanics of power embedded in medical knowledge. While inevitably more marginal than Zola's *La débâcle* since they represent, in effect, subaltern counterdiscourses, these novels are nevertheless canonical in their own way, and their dual inscription is a crucial dimension of their strategies to destabilize dominant systems of representations.

Journal du voleur, published in 1949, was Genet's first book to be released by the prestigious Gallimard publishing house. It allowed him to reach a wider and more mainstream audience than his earlier, more confidential work could ever have done. From that point on, Genet enjoyed the paradoxical privilege of being something like a sanctioned model of difference, that is an author defined simultaneously in terms of difference and sameness. Hervé Guibert's *A l'ami qui ne m'a pas sauvé la vie* (1990) and *Le protocole compassionnel* (1991), also published by Gallimard, are both the first AIDS testimonial novels and the first of Guibert's books to have become widely successful in France. Guibert, like Genet before him, became familiar to the mainstream public while also remaining radically apart from it;[9] the wide dissemination of their photographic portraits—which is not all that common for literary authors—made each of them objects of both desire and fear.[10] These three novels, written by two unapologetic, openly homosexual authors who became public sensations and celebrated writers almost overnight, are landmarks of post–World War II French literature, and their ambiguous position as both marginalized and canonical makes them particularly significant in dealing with issues of sameness and otherness in modern French culture.

Finally, I return in my conclusion to the status of communities in a universalist nation, to show how the way France has thought and fought the AIDS epidemic has been caught up from the very start in competing definitions of Frenchness.

1

Degeneracy and Inversion

The Male Homosexual as Internal Other

Much has been written on the role played by nineteenth-century medical discourses in the construction of otherness. For most cultural critics and historians of the period, post-Enlightenment otherness is an ontological category to be embodied by a variety of "Others," usually sexual or racial, and all more or less equivalent to one another thanks to their dichotomous relationship to sameness. From that perspective, otherness can alternately take the form of a "Jew," an "invert," an "Oriental," an "African," and, in France, a "German," and so on, according to the various ways that national and cultural anxieties may be played out in given historical circumstances. All "Others," then, would appear to be interchangeable signifiers.[1] In France, however, Third Republic culture presents us with a more nuanced picture of otherness, one that was determined in large part by contested and opposing views of the Republic itself. While the figure of the "Jew" came to represent a radical, viral Other in nationalist antirepublican rhetoric, that of the "homosexual" reflected universalist Enlightenment values by imagining otherness as an internally produced (but equally threatening) process of becoming rather than as an ontological entity. In the second half of the nineteenth century, the ubiquitous discourse of *dégénérescence*—meaning both "degeneracy" and "degeneration"—provided a metaphorical network along which to elaborate notions of sameness and otherness that are still operative in contemporary France.

The Discourse of *Dégénérescence*

Although it appeared also in German, English, and Italian scientific literatures, the concept of degeneration was nowhere as crucial as it was in France. Its influence was felt at all levels of French society, permeating all discourses and all politics. Malleable, filled with contradictions and inconsistencies, the concept of *dégénérescence* was used to analyze the most disparate social phenomena, and to justify their political solutions. It was used on the Left as well as on the Right, and its evolution followed the course of history, adapting to new social and political trends. Its period of maximum influence in France can be situated roughly between 1848 and 1918; to some, this central role of *dégénérescence* in the emerging field of psychiatry may explain the long resistance of French psychiatrists to Freud's theories. As Antony Copley writes: "The French psychiatrists were too strongly wedded to the achievements of their own physiological psychology to recognize any greater authority in psychoanalysis."[2]

The idea of *dégénérescence,* of course, existed before 1848. (Its origin can be traced back to Buffon and the natural sciences in the eighteenth century.) Its language also survived after World War I and was incorporated with terrifying results into totalitarian rhetoric, both on the Left and the Right. Whereas "serious" medical science abandoned almost all references to *dégénérescence* after Auschwitz, its power on the popular imagination has remained such that a concept and a rhetoric once thought of as obsolete, and fundamentally suspect, have reappeared with a vengeance in the era of AIDS, as we shall see later.

In 1857, Bénédict Augustin Morel published in Paris the first capital text on degeneration: *Traité des dégénérescences physiques, intellectuelles et morales de l'espèce humaine.* Its central idea was oddly modeled on the myth of original sin and the fall from grace, a myth "confirmed," so to speak, by the most recent advances in modern science and philosophy. While degeneration theorists did not seek explicitly to confirm religion through science, such correspondence between the underlying narrative structures of theological and scientific discourses shows the nineteenth-century bourgeois tendency to secularize existing beliefs. A degenerate, then, was a person who had lost or was in the process of losing the perfect qualities of the original type. As Morel writes:

The existence of a primitive type which the human mind likes to construct in its thinking as the masterpiece and summary of Creation, is another fact so consistent with our beliefs, that the idea of a degeneration of our nature is inseparable from the idea of a deviation from this primitive type that carried within itself the elements of the continuity of the species. These facts . . . have received today the triple approval of revealed truth, philosophy, and natural history.

[L'existence d'un type primitif que l'esprit humain se plaît à constituer dans sa pensée comme le chef-d'oeuvre et le résumé de la création, est un autre fait si conforme à nos croyances, que l'idée d'une dégénérescence de notre nature est inséparable de l'idée d'une déviation de ce type primitif, qui renfermait en lui-même les éléments de la continuité de l'espèce. Ces faits . . . de nos jours ont reçu la triple sanction de la vérité révélée, de la philosophie, et de l'histoire naturelle. (1–2)][3]

The last sentence of this passage, in particular, summarizes fairly well the evolution of Western thought since the eighteenth century: from the theological explanation to the scientific explanation of the world; it also announces the metaphorical deployment that such a concept, already metaphorical in its postulate, would soon allow. What is meant by *dégénérescence,* with and beyond Morel, is the idea of pathological changes at all levels, both individual and collective, and within a coherent movement whose telos is sterility and death—of the individual as well as the race.[4] The language of degeneration thus came to produce its own narrative, an increasingly metaphorical and self-referential narrative as signifieds tend to blur and disappear altogether. As Daniel Pick rightly remarks: "Although deployed by medical authorities, the terms were always slipping out of focus, leading into one another, crossing borderlines, signifying only another signifier. . . . *Dégénérescence* was more than just another mental condition . . . it became indeed the condition of conditions, the ultimate signifier of pathology" (8). He later adds: "Degeneration slides over from a description of disease or degradation as such, to become a kind of self-reproducing pathological process . . . which engendered a cycle of historical and social decline" (22). This is an accurate observation, but one which needs to be carried one step further: inasmuch as *dégénérescence* was a rhetorical (metaphorical) construct from the outset, it is in fact the language of *dégénérescence* which became a self-reproducing process: degeneration generating entire stories.

Under the same label, Morel and his successors gathered all sorts of pathological conditions and symptoms: cretins, albinos, consumptives, perverts of all kinds, dwarfs, deaf-mutes, criminals, prostitutes, alcoholics, et cetera. *Dégénérescence,* in its ubiquitous power, soon became the quasi-universal explanation of all the ills and evils of modern society, and all the more powerfully so since it was inscribed in a historical context in which scientific discourse had gained the increasingly hegemonic status described earlier, a status automatically granted to Morel and others.

In addition, the discourse of *dégénérescence* also participated in a larger bourgeois discourse in search of definition and legitimacy. Degeneration raised, for example, the question of hereditary transmission—an ambiguous question for a social class that had just overthrown a regime based precisely on heredity but that now needed some form of heredity in order to ensure its own political survival. *Dégénérescence* also questioned the idea of progress by suggesting the possible existence of its darker side, that is of a reverse teleological movement.[5] Mainly, *dégénérescence* provided a scientific basis to sort out who had a place and who didn't within the new society.

As soon as the French bourgeoisie seized power, the question of heredity became central to its preoccupations. As Jean Borie writes: "The constitutional arguments taking place in the various assemblies from 1789 to 1793 were organized against the principles of the monarch's heredity, against the hereditary privileges of the nobility" ["Les combats constitutionnels qui occupèrent les assemblées de 1789 à 1793 furent conduits contre le principe de l'hérédité du monarque, contre les privilèges héréditaires de la classe noble"].[6] In Borie's analysis, this revolutionary component of the bourgeoisie was, at the same time, what allowed it to seize power and what may in time prevent it from keeping it. After the revolutions of 1789, 1830, and 1848 the bourgeoisie imperatively needed to put a halt to its own revolutionary dynamics, now a threat to its power position; hence the need to naturalize the idea of transmission in order to strengthen bourgeois hegemony with the undeniability of objective, scientific facts, as well as to provide the new ruling class with a linear, teleological narrative structure. No longer based on divine right but rather on science, the new society could steadily advance toward perfection.

Yet, to this new, scientific narrative of heredity corresponds a reverse narrative, a negative one, pointing not only toward the death of individuals but also toward the extinction of the species.[7] *Dégénérescence* appears to be something like a side effect of progress, industrialization, urbanization, loosening morality, feminist ideas—in a word, of modernity. This parallel narrative provided explanations of the most traumatic crises in contemporary French society: if Napoleon III's Second Empire led to the disaster of 1870, it was because its development had been the reverse of that of the First Empire: Napoleon III was a degenerate; France's alarmingly low birthrate was a sign of the global degeneracy of the race and national community; the Paris Commune was not a romantic outburst of revolutionary fervor but one long, destructive orgy led by debauched alcoholics. The medical model in general, and the multifarious theory of *dégénérescence* in particular, would then provide a way to understand and remedy the most disconcerting social and historical phenomena.

As its field of investigation widened to cover almost all domains of human activity, medical discourse began to produce an extraordinary amount of terminology. To be sure, doctors now had to name all the new disorders resulting from recent social developments such as industrialization and the growth of cities, as well as increasing contacts with colonized populations. As they ceased to be sins and progressively became disorders, some older behaviors would also have to be renamed, for until now they had not fallen within the competence of medicine.

The linguistic inflation that took place during the second half of the nineteenth century allowed language to adapt to the new paradigm, and all these signs not only reflect a new way of seeing and conceiving the world in terms of Same and Other, but also contributed to establishing a society articulated according to this model. Indeed this dichotomous vision-conception, paralleled in medical discourse with the notions of health and pathology, would structure bourgeois language and ensure its performativity. Who belonged and who did not belong in this imagined society was decided within language. In the second half of the nineteenth century, the place of the Same and that of the Other—that is, for the latter, prisons, hospitals, psychiatric institutions, and so on, but also colonies or the other side of the Rhine—could only be constructed and distributed as such by the bar (/) that structures the Same/Other dichotomy. The performativity—and, in this case, normativity—of this discourse was its direct result. The new signifiers of health and pathology did not reflect any actual referents; rather they identified as Same or Other any element perceived as desirable or undesirable by the community: they invented and cemented ontological categories. This dual movement of inclusion and exclusion was especially efficient because biomedical discourse, as I have said, now occupied a structuring position in competition with a somewhat weakened theological discourse. Like theology, although it claimed the contrary under the cloak of empiricism, biomedical science first proposed a global explanation of nature, and then made nature conform to it. Just as vicissitudes of the soul occupy a central position in the theological paradigm, behavioral "problems," or nervous diseases, became from then on the privileged object of the new master discourse. What used to be diabolical yesterday became pathological today, that is, human. The task of identifying and excluding the pathological became particularly crucial now that the Other was so close in nature to the Same. There was but a "/" between them. The notion of sexual pathology precisely reveals the fundamental instability of this border, and, therefore, of the whole paradigm.

Inventing the Male "Homosexual"

Late-nineteenth-century medical science laid a special emphasis on pathologies of the will and of sexuality, both being inextricably linked as they equally threatened the imperviousness of the border, or the bar. Neurasthenia and abulia (or male hysteria, as it was sometimes called), the two main diseases of the will, were characterized by the loss of certain faculties associated with manliness: moral strength, physical activity, analytical skills, and the ability to make decisions, to name a few.[8] The neurasthenic or the abulic were described as impressionable, hypersensitive, abnormally receptive to raw facts rather than reasoning, subject to sudden and unexplained mood swings, going from total inaction to uncontrolled outbursts of activity. They fell prey to unrestrained imagination, and everything about them was both lacking and excessive. In a word, these men exhibited the pathological symptoms of femininity. At the time, hysteria (from the Greek *hustera,* womb, which also gave us the word "uterus") was indeed conceived as a pathological state affecting only women, the Other. In *Ventriloquized Bodies* Janet Beizer remarks that "When hysteria was attributed to men, it retained its identity as a female complaint. As a male affliction, it was usually ascribed to the effeminacy of the victim or of his life-style" (6). A man suffering from abulia could only be degenerating, since the passage from masculine to feminine was automatically seen as a regression.

Before considering male homosexuality, which was the logical outcome of nervous weakness in men, it must be noted that the nervous degenerate type is not entirely located within the new paradigm described by Laqueur.[9] Until the end of the nineteenth century, the idea of *dégénérescence* implied an internal process of degradation, or dysfunction, death being the ultimate result of completed *dégénérescence.* The feminization of men was inscribed within that process and, therefore, did not provide the stable basis of radical otherness. Feminization, then, did not constitute a radical change in ontological categories so much as a regressive change in degree, which places it closer to Laqueur's older one-sex model. Male homosexuality, for instance, was thought to come in a wide array

of levels, degrees, and intermediate stages within a process of negative development. The distinction is crucial, for the figure of the male homosexual in the
rhetoric that medicalized him did not yet represent a separate and autonomous
Other, but rather Otherness as becoming. The late-nineteenth-century male homosexual, as I will attempt to show, constituted the locus where two competing
paradigms intersected.

The term "homosexual" appeared for the first time in Germany in 1869 when
it was coined by Hungarian writer Karoly Maria Benkert. Originally meant to be
a more tolerant alternative to the morally tainted "sodomite," it was soon incorporated into medical terminology. The first and immediate consequence was the
coinage of the word "heterosexual." With this rhetorical move, sexuality became
medicalized, and articulated in terms of health and pathology. "Homosexuality"
thus became the signifier for all pathological, that is, unnatural, nonreproductive, sexuality. For Ed Cohen:

> The words "heterosexual and "homosexual" have always signified much
> more than just scientific descriptions of sexual practices. Even in its ini-
> tial usage, "homosexual" was defined exclusively as the absence of a "nat-
> ural reproductive instinct" that was supposed to direct desire toward the
> "opposite sex," while "heterosexual" was coined by symmetry to denote
> the "healthy" result that medical treatment should produce in the "patho-
> logical" male. . . . "homosexual" came to imply a type of man . . . who
> negated normal "sexual instinct," while conversely "heterosexual" re-
> deemed the pathological type by confirming the "naturalness" of the
> norm.[10]

The main medical writings on sexuality at the time, and in particular what
would become the most famous of them all, Richard von Krafft-Ebing's *Psychopathia Sexualis* (1886), seem to agree on one thing: the male homosexual represented the central figure around which all pathological sexuality gravitated
and converged in a centripetal spiral of sickness and degeneracy (and the very
idea of pathological sexuality was readily accepted at a time when syphilis was
making a dramatic comeback).[11] In this context, homosexuality provided a far
better model than masturbation, the eighteenth-century emblem of unwholesome sexuality. Masturbation was far too common a practice to be anything
more than a bad habit contracted by fundamentally normal people. In the new
paradigm structured by the dichotomy of normality and pathology, masturbation could not be a mark of otherness. In the second half of the nineteenth century, it was the excessive practice of masturbation that was thought to be pathological and, therefore, a symptom of homosexuality or predisposition to it.[12]

For Michel Foucault, in *History of Sexuality,* this move inscribed itself within the logic of the epistemological shift brought about by the Enlightenment, and the newly created homosexual became an ontological category:

> The nineteenth-century homosexual became a personage, a past, a case history, and a childhood, in addition to being a type of life, a life form, and a morphology, with an indiscreet anatomy and possibly a mysterious physiology. Nothing that went into his total composition was unaffected by his sexuality. . . . It was everywhere present in him. . . . written immodestly on his face and body. . . . It was consubstantial with him, less as a habitual sin than as a singular nature. . . . The sodomite had been a temporary aberration; the homosexual was now a species. (43)

> [L'homosexuel du XIXème siècle est devenu un personnage: un passé, une histoire et une enfance, un caractère, une forme de vie; une morphologie aussi, avec une anatomie indiscrète et peut-être une physiologie mystérieuse. Rien de ce qu'il est au total n'échappe à sa sexualité. . . . Elle lui est consubstantielle, moins comme un péché d'habitude que comme une nature singulière. . . . Le sodomite était un relaps, l'homosexuel est maintenant une espèce. (59)]

To a large extent, Foucault's description is correct. Nineteenth-century empirical medicine, to which sexuality was now answerable, tried to read all the signs of the homosexual's effeminacy on his body. Clinical descriptions of cases of homosexuality paid particular attention to the conformation of the larynx, the width of the hips, the pitch of the voice—that is, nongenital loci of femaleness.

Yet, this search for signs was far from being coherent. France's most famous nineteenth-century forensic scientist, Ambroise Tardieu, focused on, among other things, physical changes occurring to the penis because of masturbation and/or anal intercourse.[13] Such acquired marks did not constitute the characteristics of a species. In fact, this disagreement among physicians concerning the origin of the homosexual's physical characteristics directly echoed a much deeper debate around the issue of homosexuality, one which is still going on today, mostly in the field of genetics: is homosexuality inborn or acquired?[14] Limiting ourselves to the second half of the nineteenth century, we can make the following remarks: on the one hand, the distinction between acquired and inborn homosexuality could simply aim at reinforcing the idea of a true homosexuality—an inborn, pathological *perversion*—by defining a false, or circumstantial homosexuality—an acquired, behavioral *perversité;*[15] on the other hand, the indecision between the two may be seen as replicating the very instability at the core of the concept of *dégénérescence* that framed the medical discourse on pathological sexuality in France at the time. The most obvious incoherence in the discourse of *dégénérescence* is that what was once acquired could progressively become an inborn trait. Social conditions could, in the long run, modify human anatomy, and through a process of contagion a bad habit contracted in boarding school might make its way into heredity. The idea of species, then, might not so unequivocally apply to the homosexual.

To be sure, Foucault is not the only one who has attempted to explain the nineteenth-century homosexual in terms of absolute difference. As I mentioned earlier, this is actually the prevailing view among scholars. For Sander Gilman: "Images of degenerate or atavistic sexuality are used to qualify the image of the Other. Such disease entities as neurasthenia are invented, by which the Other's illness is sexual degeneracy. The sense that such illnesses are inherent in a separate class of the Other and stand apart from the normal is seen in the labeling of such diseases as inherited, and therefore outside the world of the observer."[16] I do not question the fact that sexual degeneracy was used to complete and reinforce the portrait of a previously identified Other—after all, the oppression of queers was not a new phenomenon in the mid-nineteenth century. What I do contest, however, is the idea that sexual degeneracy could be in itself a vector of radical otherness. The homosexual was not yet the Other; he was somewhere in the process of becoming the Other. Like the neurasthenic or the abulic who preceded him, he represented indecisiveness at the border between masculine and feminine. For late-nineteenth-century doctors, "true" homosexuality resulted from a pathological gender inversion of the desiring subject: a woman's soul trapped inside a man's body. The fear generated by homosexuality was not the fear of becoming a homosexual per se but rather the fear of becoming a woman. In this respect, it is especially significant that virile men who engaged in sex with other men, while supposedly retaining the "active," anally insertive position, were widely regarded as circumstantial, or false, homosexuals, not as inverts. The figure of the ("true" or "passive" or anally receptive) homosexual, therefore, was not so much a fixed category as it was a movement, a sign of gender indecision: the Same becoming Other; hence the inherent instability of inversion. In late-nineteenth-century France, "passive" homosexuality was no longer perceived as a reprehensible, libertine behavior, but neither was it perceived as a fully autonomous ontological category. Because he could not be easily reified and expelled, the invert threatened the foundations of the bourgeois nation-state from the inside, as a peril generated by the community itself—unlike the Jew, who, according to anti-Semites, was allowed in by some misplaced benevolence.

Indeed, whereas "unassimilated" Jews reproduced among themselves, it was heterosexuals who begot homosexuals one way or the other: either by means of physical degeneracy in the case of born homosexuals, or by moral degeneracy. Using the terminology presented in my general introduction, we can conclude that the theories medicalizing homosexuality in terms of degeneracy exemplify a totalizing conception of medicine, and not a localizationist one—as opposed to, say, biological anti-Semitism. Whereas the Jew was constructed essentially as a foreign body, a virus, the homosexual degenerate was seen as a product of a dysfunctioning body politic, of an internal imbalance. Moreover, considering the inherent tendency in the discourse of *dégénérescence* to reverse causes and effects, homosexuality was said to result from an overall degradation of society but also to cause that degradation. The homosexual, then, found himself twice determined, and was held responsible for a disorder of which he was also an outcome.

The danger represented by sexual inversion was especially great since its very existence seemed to question the naturalized Same/Other dichotomy which grounded the new bourgeois paradigm. Thanks to the authority of a scientific discourse constructed as the neutral vector of objective truths, the division of sexes into two distinct species—Laqueur's two-sex model—legitimated a system largely based on the separation of labor, a separation which, as George L. Mosse notes, also structured the social and sexual life of the nation.[17] On a more trivial level, homosexuality also meant sterility and wasted energy, a very serious concern in the late nineteenth century, as France was obsessed with its declining birthrate.[18] While the *ancien régime,* too, was based on the heterosexual structure of the hereditary transmission of power, this affected only the aristocracy. In the bourgeois nation-state, however, future prosperity and hold on power depended as much on the reproduction of the working (and fighting) masses as on the transmission of wealth. Heterosexuality was no longer the motor of the clan alone, but that of the whole nation. Significantly, after the disaster of 1870, it was against Germany's perceived health that France would measure its own degradation.

It is in this specific context that we must understand the extraordinary popularity the concept of *dégénérescence* and the figure of the homosexual enjoyed.[19] Until the 1890s, when a wave of right-wing nationalism began to swell and the focus on the Jew consigned the homosexual to a supporting role, the latter remained the central figure in a discourse whose entire purpose was to identify an internal cause for the national collapse. In a context which conceptualized *dégénérescence* as consubstantial to progress, the degenerate represents the

Same-Other, the Same becoming Other. The homosexual, an undecidable figure, hesitating at the border between masculine and feminine, perfectly illustrates this concept.

Literature as Medicine, or Medicine as Literature?

In his preface to the second edition of *Thérèse Raquin,* his first major success, Emile Zola expounded his theory of the naturalist novel as a reply to the critics who had accused him of immorality. The novelist, he claims, must be like a doctor who observes certain phenomena and methodically writes down what he sees. As Zola explains:

> [M]y goal was primarily scientific. . . . Read the novel carefully, and you shall see that each chapter is a curious case study in physiology. In a word, I only had one desire: . . . to write down scrupulously the feelings and actions of these human beings. I simply did on two living bodies the analytical work that surgeons do on corpses.

> [[M]on but a été un but scientifique avant tout. . . . Qu'on lise le roman avec soin, on verra que chaque chapitre est l'étude d'un cas curieux de physiologie. En un mot, je n'ai eu qu'un désir: . . . noter scrupuleusement les sensations et les actes de ces êtres. J'ai simplement fait sur deux corps vivants le travail analytique que les chirurgiens font sur les cadavres. (*Oeuvres complètes,* vol. 1, 520)]

Later in his career, Zola further developed his theories in a longer essay entitled *Le roman expérimental* (*The Experimental Novel*), in which he systematized the idea that the novel should adopt the scientific method of modern medicine and attempt to cure society of its various ills.

In *Le roman expérimental,* Zola proposes to read the theories of physiologist Claude Bernard, founder of what the latter termed "experimental medicine," to establish the basis of a new language and a new literature. Zola's approach is fairly simple: he encourages the experimental novelist to adapt to the methods of modern science, and specifically of modern medicine, to create a healthy, truthful language, and to contribute, along with other disciplines, to the betterment of the community. Zola quotes entire passages from Claude Bernard's *In-*

troduction à l'étude de la médecine expérimentale (1865), and proposes to "replace the word 'doctor' by the word 'novelist,' to clarify [his] thinking and bring to it the rigor of scientific truth" ["remplacer le mot 'médecin' par le mot 'romancier,' pour rendre [sa] pensée claire et lui apporter la rigueur d'une vérité scientifique" (*Oeuvres complètes,* vol. 10, 1175)]. And later: "Here again, just change the words 'experimental doctor' for the words 'experimental novelist,' and the whole passage applies exactly to our naturalist literature" ["Il n'y a encore ici qu'à changer les mots de médecin expérimentateur par ceux de romancier expérimentateur, et tout ce passage s'applique exactement à notre littérature naturaliste" (1189)]. And again later: "Once again, use the word 'novel' instead of the word 'medicine' and the passage remains true" ["Mettez ici encore le mot 'roman' à la place du mot 'médecine' et le passage reste vrai" (1196)].

Zola's endeavor seems to represent an attempt to validate literary discourse by giving it the power medical discourse had acquired during the second half of the nineteenth century. Literary discourse, by modeling its language on that of an exact and increasingly prestigious science, could be conceived as a neutral carrier of objective truth. In theory, realistic language should proceed by means of metonymies and spread "horizontally" to cover the largest possible field of investigation. Rhetoric would simply duplicate the inductive methods of experimental sciences. But this is, in fact, an impossible goal since it is based on a false premise. As I have already discussed, scientific discourse is itself structured by metaphors. Just like the scientific language he transposes into literature, Zola's language is grounded in metaphor, moving further from a reality it attempts to dominate and closer to the myths it hopes to eliminate.

Moreover, if the pairing of the two terms of an analogy entails the modification of both through a process of semantic contamination, medical discourse, too, becomes contaminated by its contact with literary discourse. In fact, many scientists of the period dissociated themselves from literary writers who claimed that their work had any scientific value. Max Nordau, in particular, was merciless with Zola.[20] Claude Bernard himself had clearly delineated the two domains. Zola's reply was that "the spectacle of a great scientist who can write is just as interesting as that of a great poet . . . he [the scientist] is on an equal footing with the poet" ["le spectacle d'un grand savant qui a su écrire est tout aussi intéressant que celui d'un grand poète . . . il demeure sur un pied d'égalité avec le poète" (1200)]. In his very project to authenticate his own language, Zola delegitimates and relativizes the language of science; indeed he reveals its metaphorical nature. For Jean Kaempfer, Zola's remark sets literature and science even further apart: "Calling Claude Bernard an artist . . . results in a wider gap between literature and science, thanks to an unexpected contribution: scientific fiction" ["Traiter Claude Bernard d'artiste . . . revient à ajouter de nou-velles douves au fossé qui sépare la littérature de la science, à augmenter leur écart de cet apport inattendu: la littérature scientifique"].[21] Kaempfer's analysis, however, falls a little short as he does not recognize the literariness of science in the first place. For him discourse is wrongly added to science when, in fact, it is always already there.

Back to *Le roman expérimental,* where Zola asks the following question: "Since medicine—originally an art—became a science, couldn't literature itself become a science, thanks to the experimental method?" ["Puisque la médecine, qui était un art, devient une science, pourquoi la littérature elle-même ne deviendrait-elle pas une science, grâce à la méthode expérimentale?" (1191)]. This dis-placement directly echoes the ones I mentioned earlier. What Zola fails to ac-knowledge is that medicine acquired the status of a scientific discipline by molding its discourse on that of physics and chemistry. By this I am not imply-ing that medical science somehow usurped its status thanks to a rhetorical trick. Medicine did achieve some dramatic breakthroughs in the nineteenth century. What I mean is that, to a large extent, the rhetorical move which allowed medicine to conceive of itself as a science allowed its advances, and not neces-sarily the other way round. The validation of medical discourse does not derive from its contact with the real, but rather from another, previously validated dis-course. And so on, and so forth:

> We have experimental chemistry and experimental physics; we shall soon have experimental physiology; even later, we shall have the experimental novel. Such progression is inevitable and its ultimate stage is easily fore-seeable today.

> ["On a la chimie et la physique expérimentales; on aura la physiologie ex-périmentale; plus tard encore, on aura le roman expérimental. C'est là une progression qui s'impose et dont le dernier terme est facile à prévoir dès aujourd'hui. (*Le roman expérimental,* 1182)]

What is the narrative structure of this "inevitable" progression? It is both metonymic, since it is linear and teleological, and metaphoric, since it consists in a succession of analogies. What, then, is its "ultimate stage"? Zola's structur-ing metaphor is really authenticated by another metaphor, and so on until the ultimate referent, reality, finally disappears, leaving only an *effet de réel.*[22] The subject of realism is realism itself.

Zola's critics do not take his scientific pretensions very seriously—how could we? Yet, there is a certain tendency to read somewhat superficially the rhetoric of mastery he develops in *Le roman expérimental*. In that essay, Zola deploys a rather systematic isotopy, with a proliferation of terms such as *se rendre maître* or *être maître* or *maîtriser* (to master; by far the most common of the list), *régler* (to rule, to regulate), *diriger* (to direct, to control), *asservir* (to enslave), *régner* (to reign), *obéir, conquête, conquérir, dominer, puissance* (power), and *force* (strength). These terms are directed at nature (in general, but also human nature) as well as the unknown. Foucault's concept of power/knowledge immediately comes to mind. Yet, Zola often destabilizes his own position, as he seems to indicate that such a Baconian (or post-theistic) view of nature subdued by man may not be an absolute rule after all. He writes, for example: "If we do not stop at the metaphysical man of the classical age, we must take into account the ideas our age has [*se fait*] about nature and life" ["Si nous n'en restons pas à l'homme métaphysique de l'âge classique, il nous faut bien tenir compte des nouvelles idées que notre âge *se fait* de la nature et de la vie" (1191; my emphasis)]. Interestingly, the French expression *se faire des idées* also means "to imagine things" or "to delude oneself." What is implied by this very telling expression is that each historical period makes—indeed, makes up—its own set of ideas. In a passage like this one, Zola unwittingly recognizes the fact that scientific knowledge is also produced by a given worldview in a given historical context—in a word, by a preexisting paradigm. Far from the universalizing ambitions of the bourgeoisie, Zola seems to entertain the theoretical possibility—or inevitability, even—of future paradigm shifts, that is, of revolutions (in the rich, Kuhnian sense of the term). If Zola could not stick to his avowed project as presented in his critical writings, it may be because he could sense its relativity. In a larger cultural sense, what Zola's theories of medicine and literature reveal and exemplify is the enduring, indeed inherent, instability at the core of constructions of sameness and otherness in modern France.

2

⟨⟩

Gender Indecision and Cultural Anxiety

Outing Zola

Do Zola's novels have any scientific value at all?[1] More specifically, can the theses propounded in *Le roman expérimental* give us any particular insight in our reading of *La débâcle,* Zola's novelization of the French defeat by Prussia in the war of 1870? While Zola's science remains largely dubious, his claims to cure social ills through the art of the novel do deserve attention for, among other things, the role of narratives in the production of a national identity. The point of this chapter, then, is not to determine whether Zola's novels are scientifically valid, but rather to examine *La débâcle* in its performative aspect. What follows attempts to show how Zola's text sways between the cultural (and textual) production of metaphors and the metaphorical production of culture (and the text), and specifically how disease metaphors are both ideological and generative.[2] For Zola the disease metaphor, and specifically the metaphor of degeneration, or *dégénérescence,* is a generative one. *Dégénérescence,* a metaphorical construct supposed to signify (the fear of) the annihilation of the great bourgeois narrative, becomes in fact the source of the author's narrative. Indeed, in Zola's text degeneration is generation. *La débâcle* articulates itself along the underlying pathological figure of the "homosexual" and, in that respect, the novel exemplifies universalist ideals. Yet Zola does not and cannot adhere unequivocally to his ideological framework. Ultimately, the text confers a large degree of narrative au-

31

thority upon a degenerate character, destabilizing both the scientific discourse supposed to authenticate the literary discourse and the healthy/unhealthy dichotomy in which such a discourse attempts to ground and naturalize its hegemonic claims. In so doing, Zola unwittingly reveals the metaphorical nature of a certain medical discourse that was on its way to acquiring an increased structural role in French society during the second half of the nineteenth century.

Theory and Practice of the Experimental Novel

At first glance, *La débâcle* appears to fit perfectly with the project of *Le roman expérimental*. Literary and scientific discourses seem to match even in the structure of the book as a whole. Critics have noted how Zola's focus, like that of a microscope, narrows itself from the large to the small, from France to the French, from the emperor to the foot soldier.[3] Such a narrative movement corresponds to that of biomedical science: Zola seeks the causes of a national catastrophe in the individuals who make up the nation, just as medicine looks for the microscopic agents of a larger pathology. In addition, the discourse of *dégénérescence,* so influential on Zola's work, reads the individual as signifier for the entire species, thus legitimating further the novelist's narrative strategy. The collapse of the community is almost entirely told in and by the individual pathological characters used simultaneously as metaphors and synecdoches.

With *La débâcle,* Zola was nearing the end of the twenty-volume Rougon-Macquart cycle, in which he told of life under the Second Empire through the history of a family. In this penultimate novel, Zola follows two main characters, two soldiers, from the last days of the Franco-Prussian War to the Paris Commune. Jean Macquart is the simple carpenter turned peasant, already introduced in an earlier novel, *La terre,* and Maurice Levasseur is a deracinated and psychologically weaker city-dweller. The two men soon become friends before being repeatedly separated and reunited during the chaotic aftermath of the defeat. Eventually, Maurice sides with the Communards, and as French troops enter Paris to crush the uprising Jean, still a soldier in the regular army, kills him without realizing who it was at first. Around the double nucleus of Jean and Maurice, representing the fracture of the national community, circulates an ensemble of secondary characters, equally symbolic of various social ills and their potential cures. To describe the men in Jean's squad, Zola uses a language of truth, that of physiological descriptions. Empirical observations and the neutral language that transcribes them uncover the deeper truth of the object being observed, that is, a moral pathology which never fails to leave its marks on the body. Tropes are not adornments but rather tools for a better intelligibility. If Loubet, one of the soldiers, resembles a fox, if Lapoulle, another soldier, has the face of a pig, it is because they are exactly that: their physical appearances remind us of these animals we have associated with certain character traits. Zola builds up quite a bestiary, in fact. One character has "the face of a well-trained dog" (3; translation modified) ["une face de bon chien" (403)], another a "lion's head" (18; translation modified) ["tête de lion" (418)].[4] To the language of *dégénérescence*, Zola adds that of Darwinism as each character's anatomy betrays the underlying narrative of his or her evolution.

Destinies of crime and perversion are inscribed on the bodies of Sambuc, Cabasse, and Ducat, the three francs-tireurs in charge of guerilla warfare against the Prussians. Cabasse exhibits his criminal tendencies: he is "tall and spare, with swarthy features and a long, blade-like nose" (115) ["grand et sec, la face noire, avec un long nez en lame de couteau" (512)]. His nose, his body even, have the shape of a blade because he is a potential murderer. The swarthiness of his face represents that of his mind and past: "An act of larceny, never quite cleared up" (116) ["toute une histoire de vol restée obscure" (513)]. (The French phrase "histoire de vol," with its double meaning, is particularly telling since *histoire* means both "story" and "history"; both meanings largely overlap in the rhetoric of *dégénérescence*, where every individual story always uncovers a deeper case history, where each anecdote summarizes a destiny.) Cabasse's accomplice, Ducat, is "short and fat, with a white face and thinning hair" (115) ["petit et gros, blême, les cheveux rares" (512)]. Everything about this man "full of Latin tags" betrays the fact that he "had once served as court bailiff in Blainville, but had been forced to resign following a number of improprieties with small girls" (116) ["ancien huissier de Blainville, forcé de vendre sa charge après des aventures malheureuses avec des petites filles" and who "citait du latin" (513)]. This social downfall of the pervert, the "déclassé" (819), is announced by his complexion, his flesh, his baldness, his false erudition. In the novel, the francs-tireurs are "cunning rascals that didn't give a damn for anybody" (413) ["des gaillards adroits qui faisaient leurs affaires en se fichant du monde" (820): literally, "were doing their business"]. Ducat, whose very name evokes money, is now an accountant who takes advantage of his position, basic education, and articulateness to corrupt little children and satisfy the unwholesome tendencies written all over his anatomy.

As for Chouteau, another soldier in Jean's squad, his portrayal corresponds to the type of the urban degenerate, the hysterical agitator who spreads moral decay across the community. He too, like Ducat, has access to language, but again a perverted and infectious language:

> He was the resident corruptor, the shoddy workman from Montmartre, this idle, roistering house-painter who—fed on the undigested scraps of speeches heard at public meetings—mingled the most outrageous rubbish with the noble principles of liberty and equality. He knew everything and was bent on indoctrinating his comrades. (38–39)

> [C'était le pervertisseur, le mauvais ouvrier de Montmartre, le peintre en bâtiment flâneur et noceur, ayant mal digéré les bouts de discours entendus dans les réunions publiques, mêlant des âneries révoltantes aux grands principes d'égalité et de liberté. Il savait tout, il endoctrinait les camarades. (437–38)]

The results are soon felt: "Loud cheers greeted his words. Corruption was taking its toll" (39) ["Des bravos éclatèrent, la perversion agissait" (438)]. Chouteau's rhetoric is disjointed and incomplete; he is unable to synthesize the fragments of discourses he has managed to pick up here and there but couldn't comprehend. His social unproductiveness logically corresponds to his inability to use the coherent language of truth and reason. From a structural standpoint, this character represents, within the fictional text, the type of language naturalist novelists criticized, for such language was considered not only the product of sick and degenerate minds but also one of the root causes of contemporary social ills.

Chouteau—and, to a lesser extent, his accomplice Loubet—reappears on several occasions during the course of the novel—even at the cost of verisimilitude, as when he resurfaces suddenly at the end among the Communards. To be more precise, if Zola keeps twisting the internal logic of the narration in order to have Chouteau return at regular intervals, it is because his symbolic role is so crucial to the novel's thesis. Chouteau represents the corrupting element that undoes the community from within, feeding off social decay, regenerating, as it were, and refusing to disappear.

As he does with Ducat, Zola seems to hesitate between two types of figures. On the one hand, Chouteau and Loubet, the bad soldiers, represent an internal disease, the degeneration of a body politic whose immune system turns against what it is supposed to guard, hence inducing its degradation. Here, Zola is still coherent with his initial project. Yet, he describes them in terms of otherness. Chouteau and Loubet do not quite correspond to the passive, self-destructive degenerate type, but rather to an active, resistant, corrupting element. Unlike the degenerate whose sterility and death figure and foreshadow that of the body politic, the foreign body survives and proliferates. With these two characters, Zola is moving away from the totalizing model, or what I called, following Cindy Patton, the immunological model, that of passive degeneracy, as he is describing with a language of radical otherness the corrupting element as foreign body.

At the end of the following excerpt, depicting hordes of foreigners coming from the East to steal from the corpses left on the battlefield, Zola finally lets out the word the whole passage seems to be leading to: *juiverie*. Understandably, the 1968 English translation I have been using does not include any such explicit reference to Jews. The 1893 translation (1914 edition, titled *The Downfall*), however, does, as it seems to revel in anti-Semitic overtones.

> Then, on perceiving some people on his left, two men and a woman, it occurred to him to question them. But the woman fled at his approach, and the men warned him away with threatening gestures. Others whom he saw, clad in sordid garments, inexpressibly filthy, and with the suspicious-looking faces of bandits, were careful to avoid him, slinking away between the bushes like crawling, crafty animals. And on noticing that the dead, in the rear of these evil-looking men, were shoeless, displaying their bare feet in the grey light, he ended by realising that these prowlers were some of the tramps following the hostile armies, plunderers of corpses, predatory German Jews, who had entered France in the wake of the invasion. One tall, thin fellow darted away ahead of him at a gallop, with a sack burdening his shoulders, and stolen silver and stolen watches jingling in his pockets. (355; 1893 translation)

> Then, catching sight of some people away to the left, two men and a woman, he decided to question them, but as soon as he approached them the woman took to her heels, and the men drove him away. He saw some more. But they, too, made off, disappearing hurriedly into the undergrowth like suspicious animals, dressed in unspeakably dirty clothes, shifty looking as poachers. Then he noticed that none of the dead bodies left behind by this shady bunch had any boots on, and realized that the wretched creatures were thieves, who followed in the wake of the German armies, preying on the wounded and stripping the corpses. One of them, a tall, thin fellow, dashed past with a sack slung over his shoulder, his pockets bulging with watches and silver coins stolen from the dead and dying. (339; 1968 translation)

[Puis, apercevant du monde à sa gauche, deux hommes et une femme, il eut l'idée de les questionner. Mais, à son approche, la femme s'enfuit, les hommes l'écartèrent du geste, menaçants; et il en vit d'autres, et tous l'évitaient, filaient entre les broussailles, comme des bêtes rampantes et sournoises, vêtus sordidement, d'une saleté sans nom, avec des faces louches de bandits. Alors, en remarquant que les morts, derrière ce vilain monde, n'avaient plus de souliers, les pieds nus et blêmes, il finit par comprendre que c'étaient là de ces rôdeurs qui suivaient les armées allemandes, des détrousseurs de cadavres, toute une basse juiverie de proie, venue à la suite de l'invasion. Un grand maigre fila devant lui en galopant, les épaules chargées d'un sac, les poches sonnantes des montres et des pièces blanches volées dans les goussets. (742–43)]

Although the 1893 translation overstates them, this passage contains unmistakable anti-Semitic elements that are downplayed in the 1968 translation.[5] Jews, at the time, were seen by some as profiting from France's weaknesses. Moreover, this entire depiction, seen through the eyes of Prosper, a secondary character, recalls the portrayals of the *Ostjuden,* the Eastern Jews, during the period.[6] Zola's opening descriptions of the French armies before the battle, waiting for the disaster to come from the East, also conjure up the mysterious fear of a fantasized Orient, a dangerous Orient which, at the time, was more often than not associated with the Jews. Consider the following excerpts: "the dark horizon . . . the whole of that purple East" (6) ["l'horizon envahi de ténèbres, tout cet Orient violâtre" (406)]; "gazing eastwards towards the Rhine, which was now completely enveloped in night—a dark wall enshrouded in mystery" (11) ["cet Orient où la nuit s'était déjà complètement faite, un mur noir assombri de mystères" (410)]; "Now, in the East, the first pallor of day was appearing; an infinitely sad, dank greyness" (19) ["Maintenant, à l'Orient, le jour blanchissait, un jour louche" (419)]; "the army was turning its back away from Paris and heading eastwards, into the unknown" (63) ["on tournait le dos à Paris, allant là-bas, vers l'est, à l'inconnu" (461)]. The Orient, here, is the land of all perils, the dark, unfathomable domain of the radical Other. And in the 1890s, the radical Other was the Jew.

The mysterious darkness surrounding the French troops, then, does remind us of the evil side of progress, as in the *dégénérescence* model. This time, it evokes and provokes the panic inspired by the unknowable Other whose presence is nowhere to be seen, yet is felt everywhere. According to this model, the community is threatened not by an internal collapse but by a virus-like entity, an enemy all the more dangerous as he is invisible: we are no longer dealing with a familiar, indeed familial disease. Zola's stylistic choices directly reflect the changing context of the late nineteenth century, which faced a recurrence of epidemic diseases such as syphilis and cholera and the discoveries of new viruses and bacteria, along with science's inability to resolve many of these problems.

The origin of this shift to a localizing (or virological) model of description, with its accompanying anti-Semitic connotations, can be found in the very plurality of *dégénérescence:* the body politic had been weakened from the inside, which made it more vulnerable to attacks from the outside. By modeling literary discourse on medical discourse, Zola inevitably incorporated into the former the latter's intertexts, postulates, contradictions, and ideology. As a result, literature exposes the poetic and superstitious dimensions of biomedical science. The anti-Semitic and orientalist descriptions mentioned above were not produced by some repressed anti-Semitism on Zola's part so much as they were inscribed in the very project of *Le roman expérimental.*

Appropriating Claude Bernard's terminology in his own essay, Zola writes, for example:

> The social *circulus* is identical to the vital *circulus:* in society, as in the human body, there exists an interdependence linking the various limbs and organs together, so that, if one organ begins to decay, several others are affected, and a very complex disease breaks out. In our novels, then, when we experiment on a serious wound poisoning society, we proceed like the experimental doctor.

> [Le *circulus* social est identique au *circulus* vital: dans la société comme dans le corps humain, il existe une solidarité qui lie les différents membres, les différents organes entre eux, de telle sorte que, si un organe se pourrit, beaucoup d'autres sont atteints, et qu'une maladie très complexe se déclare. Dès lors, dans nos romans, lorsque nous expérimentons sur une plaie grave qui empoisonne la société, nous procédons comme le médecin expérimentateur. (1189)]

With this metaphorical translation from medical to literary discourse, Zola thinks he is only borrowing the doctor's analytical method—"we proceed *like*"— when he is also appropriating and reproducing its founding ideology—we proceed *with.* Zola, therefore, will not and cannot identify on his own any "complex disease" or "serious wound" or their causes: all this is provided to him by a normative discourse that has already identified, that is, performed, the pathological categories Zola will reuse as is. With this I am not implying that Claude

Bernard's theories are anti-Semitic; on the contrary, his emphasis on the *milieu intérieur* fits the model of totalizing medicine I presented earlier, a model in which viruses and other ontological bodies play little or no part. What I mean to say is that Zola himself may not be so discriminating. As he emulates biomedical discourse in general, he does not differentiate among its various internal tendencies, incompatible as they may be.

In the specific case of *La débâcle,* the reader could expect Germany to represent the Other, the virus. Actually Zola remains within his initial project, as depictions of Germany's health allow him to present what really preoccupies him, France's internal illness. In the opening pages of the novel, he describes the German army as a healthy body whose brain is in possession of all its faculties and allows the good functioning of all limbs and organs. Enemy soldiers, often depicted as ants or locusts, are not like viruses or pathogenic elements attacking a previously healthy body, but rather, in a Darwinian perspective, a fitter species in the struggle for life. Germany is a model. In contrast, France is described in terms of internal imbalance and advanced degeneracy. Echoing the above excerpt from *Le roman expérimental,* the French army represents a perfect case. It is affected in its two structuring axes, in its hierarchy as well as in the relations among soldiers, and is ultimately, "under the leadership of the Emperor, sick and vacillating, duping himself and duping others" (113) ["l'empereur à leur tête, souffrant et hésitant, trompé et se trompant" (413); literally, "deceived by some and making mistakes"], like a diseased brain. Beyond the army, it is the future of France that was already inscribed in the narrative structure of *dégénérescence* underlying all descriptions of degenerates in medical texts. Borrowing their rhetoric, Zola accepts its telos: "France bewildered, left in disarray, retarded and perverted, lacking the necessary leaders, men, and arms. And the horrible prediction was coming true" (my translation) ["La France effarée, livrée au désordre, attardée et pervertie, n'ayant ni les chefs, ni les hommes, ni les armes nécessaires. Et l'affreuse prédiction se réalisait" (559)].

In *Feux et signaux de brume: Zola,* Michel Serres emphasizes the kinship not only among some of the characters in *La débâcle* but also between France and Germany. There is, for instance, the pairing of cousin Gunther and Goliath, the Prussian spy (two minor characters) with whom Silvine (another minor character) had a son. If we consider the synecdoche making the individual stand for the whole species, one can easily deduce the nations' kinship from the characters', and Serres can rightly remark: "Let's leave . . . the individual aside, it is only a small-scale model," ["Laissons . . . l'individuel, il n'est que modèle réduit" (310)], and conclude that "[t]he Prussians are also part of the Rougon-Macquarts" ["Les Prussiens sont aussi quelques Rougon-Macquart" (314)]. From this perspective, Serres reinscribes *La débâcle* within a hereditary narrative that goes beyond the Rougon-Macquart cycle: "As if . . . corrupt Latins and German saviors . . . were produced by the same tree, or born from the same ancestors. As if the stock of the Rougon-Macquarts was generalized suddenly to include Europe, the Indo-European tree" ["Comme si . . . Latins corrompus et Germains sauveurs . . . étaient produits par le même arbre, ou issus des mêmes ancêtres. Comme si la souche des Rougon-Macquart se généralisait, tout à coup, à l'Europe, à l'arbre indo-européen" (318)]. Serres's analysis is particularly interesting in that it explains why Germany is often depicted in positive terms in the novel, in opposition to the downward logic of the *dégénérescence* metaphor, yet along the same underlying axis, that of heredity. Germany and France appear to be two relatives, one who succeeded, one who degenerated. However, some questions remain unanswered in Serres's essay. Why these two opposing evolutions? And, more important, when and why did these rival brothers—*frères ennemis* as Serres calls them—become enemies? Darwinism may help but it could also raise as many questions as it answers. The fact is that, once again, Zola seems unable to adopt a single, coherent scientific explanation by which he might authenticate his narrative.

In addition, the line between health and disease is not just the Rhine. On the French side, some characters, such as Jean, Maurice's sister Henriette, and the military surgeon symbolize the community's power of regeneration. If the disease is internal, so is its cure. The soil of France, the land, reminds us that such regeneration is always possible, it is the ultimate point of reference. The health of the characters, and therefore of the community, is measured by their relation to the land, a gendered, heterosexual relation. Zola frequently uses the adjective "fertile" to describe the plains and the fields. In turn, Henriette who, unlike her brother, stayed in the countryside, is described in terms that link her directly to the land. Her blond hair, Zola insists, is like "ripe oats" ["avoine mûre"]. In her relation to the wounded soldiers in her care, her maternal role represents something of a national ideal: Henriette is also like the mother of the country, the *mère patrie*. To describe the inner workings of her emotions—Henriette feels, of course, she does not think—Zola uses a metaphor that complements the mother/land metaphor:

> Her heart was still ravaged . . . ; and if now she was beginning to experience some assuagement, some new tenderness, she was completely unaware of it; what was happening to her was as imperceptible as the subtle modifications that take place in a germinating seed, a process that remains invisible to the closest observer. She was even unaware of the pleasure she derived from the hours spent at Jean's bedside. (404–5)

[Son coeur restait meurtri; et s'il y entrait un soulagement, une tendresse nouvelle, ce ne pouvait être qu'à son insu: tout un de ces sourds cheminements de la graine qui germe, sans que rien, au regard, révèle le travail caché. Elle ignorait jusqu'au plaisir qu'elle avait fini par prendre à rester des heures près du lit de Jean. (812)]

The feelings she is beginning to have for Jean, the peasant, are entirely passive on her part: another is planting the seed. Jean is both the one who cultivates the fields and the one who allows the woman to authenticate herself through her relation to the land. For Zola, just as all disorder comes from a dysfunctioning heredity, that is, from a heterosexual process gone awry, health is figured by metaphors of fertility and motherhood. Health is not wilderness or "natural nature," as symbolized by the horses (and some soldiers) left to themselves and their most destructive instincts, but rather nature that has been domesticated and is entirely governed by its reproductive function. In a word, health is heterosexuality.

The military surgeon, major Bouroche, provides us with yet another model of masculinity. The particular relevance of this character lies in the fact that he also represents the naturalist novelist within the text; his task is similar to the one Zola assigned to himself. The very first time Bouroche appears in the novel, he delineates immediately everyone's places and attributions within the heterosexual order he rules. A step-by-step reading of the scene reveals the ideological, hetero-normative frame in which Zola inscribes the figure of the doctor. In the beginning of the passage, the village crowd is left to itself after the departure of the man whose declining authority failed to keep it under control, Marshal MacMahon, commander in chief of the French army. "Bareheaded and half undressed" (218) ["nu-tête, à moitié dévêtu" (615)], MacMahon appears diminished in his virility, as he is grotesquely wounded in the buttocks. This strategically placed wound—and the "vague expression in his eyes" (218–19) ["il regardait, d'un air vague" (615)], a direct echo of the sick emperor's empty gaze—symbolically betrays his inability to fulfill the duties of his position of power: the regime's failure is inscribed on the body of its army's commander— to be specific, on his ass.

As we have seen, late-nineteenth-century psychology constructed crowds in terms of femininity: crowds were thought to be irrational and subject to unrestrained imagination. In a word, they needed a master. With the departure of MacMahon, taken away in a wagon, the position of power is left vacant. The frightened crowd is kept in the dark and starts producing its own (false) knowledge of the situation with rumors and exaggerations, that is, a disorderly mode of discourse.[7] A new type of man must make his entrance and assume power.

Symbolically, the fog clears and the sun comes out to announce the arrival of this new man, the man of science, who will restore both the social order and the order of discourse:

> Near the Place du Collège the waggon disappeared amongst the increasing crowd, amongst whom the most extraordinary stories about the battle were circulating. The fog had cleared, and the streets were filled with sunlight. (219)

> [Vers la place du collège, la carriole qui emportait le maréchal, se perdait au milieu de la foule grossie, parmi laquelle circulaient déjà les plus extraordinaires nouvelles du champ de bataille. Le brouillard se dissipait, les rues s'emplissaient de soleil. (616)]

The man's presence is first felt as a rough, hence masculine, voice, giving orders to be obeyed without question. Unlike the women who make up most of the crowd, and who remedy their ignorance of the situation with irrational fantasies and false knowledge, the doctor uses language to restore order. And the first thing this language orders is that the women return inside, to the private sphere they had left so that they could participate, nonproductively and hysterically, in the public debate. As for the man, he will rid himself of the discredited symbol of authority, his military uniform, to put on the outfit of the man of science:

> But someone in the courtyard shouted roughly: "It's not out there you're needed, ladies, but in here!" The three women returned to the yard, where they found Major Bouroche, who had already thrown his uniform into a corner and put on a large white apron. (219)

> [Mais une voix rude cria de la cour: —Mesdames, ce n'est pas dehors, c'est ici qu'on a besoin de vous! Elles rentrèrent toutes trois, elles se trouvèrent devant le major Bouroche qui avait déjà jeté dans un coin son uniforme, pour revêtir un grand tablier blanc. (616)]

Bouroche's authority is further suggested by his name—*roche* or "rock": Bouroche is solid, unmoved, impassible, in perfect contrast with the confused women. Once inside:

> With his enormous head, his wiry, bristling hair, his snub-nosed, lion-like face gleaming with energy, and, above all, that huge, still spotless apron, he presented such a terrifying appearance that all of sudden they belonged to him and were only too ready to do anything he asked them, almost knocking one another down in their efforts to please him. (219; translation modified)

[Sa tête énorme aux durs cheveux hérissés, son mufle de lion flambait de hâte et d'énergie, au-dessus de toute cette blancheur, encore sans tache. Et il leur apparut si terrible qu'elles lui appartinrent du coup, obéissant à un signe, se bousculant pour le satisfaire. (616)]

The lion metaphor in the original French conjures up the image of the male among the females, thus legitimating the distribution of sexual roles by naturalizing it. As for "toute cette blancheur encore sans tache," it calls to mind the whiteness of the sheets before being soiled by the deflowering (as well as the blank page on which a new discourse may be written; but both images are, I think, linked). Bouroche's haste and energy are similar to that of the man about to consummate his marriage, as emphasized by the sexual connotations of the verb "belong." Women are there "to please him." Thus, with the sole authority of his voice, the doctor has restored order, a phallic, heterosexual order.

I mentioned earlier that the character of the surgeon allowed Zola to be present in his text. This correspondence is first suggested by their common usage of authoritative/authorial language to order and distribute roles. In a more metaphoric way, the amputation scenes are equally telling. Bouroche does to the soldiers' bodies what Zola advocates for French society in his theories of the novel. Both the surgeon and the experimental novelist identify, then amputate the rotten limbs that threaten to infect the whole body. Both face heroically the horror around them, devoted as they are to their cleansing mission. The following passage about Bouroche performing amputations reveals Zola's ideas on his own role as novelist:

But, completely preoccupied, breathless with exhaustion, he merely went on with his work, paying no attention to anybody. He was talking to himself, half aloud, counting them, giving them numbers, classifying them: this one first, next that one, then that one over there; a jawbone, an arm, a thigh. (273)

[Mais lui, tout à son affaire, soufflant de lassitude, organisait son travail, sans écouter personne. Il se parlait à voix haute, il les comptait du doigt, leur donnait des numéros, les classait: celui-ci, celui-là, puis cet autre; un, deux, trois; une mâchoire, un bras, une cuisse. (674)]

Zola's rhetoric has come full circle, as the amputation scenes in the novel are a metaphor for a metaphor, that is, for Zola's own metaphor of amputation in *Le roman expérimental.*

As for the (pro)creative virility of the naturalist author according to Zola, it appeared explicitly a few years later in his reply to a man who accused him of having plagiarized his novel *Rome:*

> I have already devoted more than thirty years of my existence to creation, and the children are there, more than a thousand came out of me. . . . Haven't I sufficiently proved my virility as a creator of men? . . . Come on, little man, you may say that I need everything, that I assimilate everything; but you will never make anyone believe that my throngs of children are not my own!

> [J'ai déjà passé plus de trente ans de mon existence à créer, et les enfants sont là, plus de mille, sortis de moi. . . . Est-ce que je n'ai point assez prouvé ma virilité de créateur d'hommes? . . . Allez, allez, petit monsieur, vous pouvez dire que j'ai besoin de tout et que je m'assimile tout; mais vous ne ferez jamais croire à personne que ma nuée d'enfants ne sont pas de moi!][8]

Zola did not invent the metaphor associating artistic creation and procreation, of course, but the distinction between male language on the one hand, and a corrupt and corrupting effeminate language on the other, between the type of new intellectual figured by Bouroche in *La débâcle* and by Doctor Pascal in *Le docteur Pascal* (the next and final novel in the Rougon-Macquart saga), and those degenerate intellectuals, false prophets of a false science, is a central tenet of Zola's project. Language, too, may be healthy or pathological, as Zola implies throughout *Le roman expérimental.*

Naturalism as Heterosexuality

Zola's primary goal was to free the novel from the yoke of Romanticism and return it to the "true" writers. In his attacks against the Romantics, he distinguished between two incompatible types of language: Romantic language, essentially effeminate, and naturalist language, masculine and heterosexual. He writes in *Le roman expérimental:* "Today we are rotting with lyricism, we wrongly believe that great style is made of sublime confusion, always about to descend into madness: great style is made of logic and clarity" ["Nous sommes actuellement pourris de lyrisme, nous croyons bien à tort que le grand style est fait d'un effarement sublime, toujours près de culbuter dans la démence: le grand style est fait de logique et de clarté" (1200)]. In what follows, Zola systematically di-

vides language between effeminacy and manliness, attributing feminine characteristics to lyricism and masculine characteristics to logic and clarity. But this
gendered opposition is complicated by the healthy/pathological dichotomy so
as to articulate, in and with language, the notion of pathological sexuality.

In his "Lettre à la jeunesse" ("A Letter to Young People"), published as part of
Le roman expérimental, Zola first acknowledges the positive contribution of Romanticism, and he describes the state of language at the beginning of the nineteenth century in thinly veiled phallic terms: "Language, weakened by three
hundred years of classical usage, was nothing more than a dull tool, without
vigor. A generation of lyrical poets was necessary to adorn it anew, to make it a
large, flexible, and shiny instrument" ["La langue, affaiblie par trois cents ans
d'usage classique, restait un outil émoussé et sans vigueur. Il fallait, je le répète,
une génération de poètes lyriques pour empanacher la langue, pour en faire un
instrument large, souple et brillant" (1210)]. Language is portrayed as a masculine instrument, and the problem with the Romantics is that they fail to use it
productively: their creative energy is wasted. From this point on, Zola develops
a metaphorical system directly based on the medical concepts of degeneration
and pathological sexuality. His descriptions of the Romantics almost literally
echo the clinical portraits of homosexuals in the medical texts of the period. In
effect, the problem with romantic literature, precisely like male homosexuality,
is that it is self-referential instead of being turned outward, toward reality.

What and who, then, is considered pathological, that is, homosexual? A literary discourse which reflects not the real but rather an unrestrained imagination; the reader who is enthused with such a discourse; and the urban intellectual who authors it. Thus, Zola writes: "To applaud a rhetoric, to become
enthused with an ideal, these are but beautiful, high-strung emotions; women
weep when they hear music. Today we need the manliness of truth" ["Applaudir
une rhétorique, s'enthousiasmer pour l'idéal, ce ne sont là que de belles émo-
tions nerveuses; les femmes pleurent quand elles entendent de la musique. Aujourd'hui, nous avons besoin de la virilité du vrai" (1206)]. And later:

> The ideal generates all sorts of dangerous dreams. . . . As soon as one
> leaves the solid ground of the real, one gets thrown among all sorts of
> monstrosities. Take for example romantic novels and drama . . . you'll find
> in them the most shameful refinements of debauchery, the most amazing
> follies of the flesh and the mind. . . . With naturalism, this hypocrisy of
> secretly arousing vices is impossible.

> [L'idéal engendre toutes les rêveries dangereuses. . . . Du moment où l'on
> quitte le terrain solide du vrai, on est lancé dans toutes les monstruosités.

Prenez les romans et les drames romantiques . . . vous y trouverez les raffinements les plus honteux de la débauche, les insanités les plus stupéfiantes de la chair et de l'esprit. . . . Avec les oeuvres naturalistes, cette hypocrisie du vice secrètement chatouillé est impossible. (1229)]

But if language can corrupt, it can also cure. Zola constructs himself as a masculine, heterosexual author, out to cure the ills of the nation (and specifically the declining birthrate of France compared to that of Germany) by cleansing language itself:

We are losing ourselves in lyrical rantings, we neglect the facts to drown in some sort of obscure ideal. This is why, when we should be at the top after tirelessly throwing the seeds of truth to the wind, we are today so diminished and crushed by heavier, more methodical races.

[Nous nous perdons en déclamations lyriques, nous dédaignons les faits pour nous noyer dans je ne sais quel idéal obscur. Voilà pourquoi, nous qui devrions être au sommet après les semences de vérité que nous avons sans cesse jetées au vent, nous sommes à cette heure amoindris, écrasés par des races plus lourdes et plus méthodiques. (1230)]

The rhetoric developed in passages such as these is systematic in *Le roman expérimental* and in Zola's other critical writings. He does not simply structure his metaphors in terms of gender but, by juxtaposing a metaphor of pathology, he adds to the equation the terms of heterosexuality/homosexuality. Beizer rightly shows how the text of the whole Rougon-Macquart cycle undermines the initial project and ultimately collapses the two terms of the dichotomy: "At roughly the same time Freud was grappling with issues of bisexuality, Zola was using sexual figures to represent what we might call tendencies toward bitextuality: that is, fantasies of hermaphroditic authorship."[9] Beizer's analysis, however, seems somewhat limited insofar as what she means by "bitextuality" is a textuality that would be both male and female, but still heterosexual. Reducing homosexuality to a subcategory within the larger question of gender could end up perpetuating its exclusion from both literary and critical discourses.

In fact, Zola raged against homosexuality, particularly as the war against Prussia loomed on the horizon. Like degeneration, thought to have a special relationship with the idea of progress, homosexuality as well was often regarded at the time as the mysterious and malevolent double of heterosexuality. Nineteenth-century medical discourse constructed sexual inversion as a pathological disorder, the undecidable, the enemy within, the destructive force produced by heterosexuality itself but which, at the same time, undid what the bourgeois nation-state was trying to build. Homosexuality, produced from within bour-geois discourse, kept reminding this discourse of the impossibility of its closure.

In his article "Au couvent" ("In the Convent"), Zola condemns all educational institutions which separate the sexes and which, according to him, foster homosexuality: "Remember secondary school. Vices grow liberally there, and one lives as in the midst of Roman decadence. All cloistered association of per-sons of the same sex is bad for morals" ["Souvenez-vous du collège. Les vices y poussent grassement, on y vit en pleine pourriture romaine. Toute association cloîtrée de personnes d'un même sexe est mauvaise pour la morale"].[10] (It seems that Zola could have applied this comment to military life. As we shall see, he should have.) In another article entitled "La fin de l'orgie" ("The End of the Orgy"), he attacks the cross-dressing debaucheries of the Sec-ond Empire:

> Truly, the empire has made a great nation out of us. Now our men are be-coming women. When Rome was rotting in her greatness, she accom-plished the very same mistakes. The beautiful nights of the ancient orgy are back, the ardent nights when humans no longer have a sex.

> [Vraiment l'empire a fait de nous une grande nation. Voilà que nos hommes deviennent des femmes. Lorsque Rome pourrissait dans sa grandeur, elle n'a pas accompli d'autres miracles. Les belles nuits de l'orgie antique sont revenues, les nuits ardentes où les créatures n'ont plus de sexe.]

And later:

> It was inevitable. When the blasé are bored, they invent some monstros-ity to entertain themselves. The empire threw so many loose girls into their arms, so many adulterous wives, that a real woman has surely be-come a scanty treat; they yawn when they look at her, they have had enough of her grace and beauty. But a woman who is a man, a dress from the right maker in which a tall, bearded fellow is enclosed, now that awak-ens the mind and tickles curiosity. Nothing's better to shake off one's sated boredom, and recover one's taste for living.

> [Ils devaient forcément en arriver là. Lorsque les blasés s'ennuient, ils in-ventent quelque monstruosité pour se distraire. L'empire leur a jeté aux bras tant de filles galantes, tant d'épouses adultères, qu'une femme véri-table est sans doute devenue pour eux un maigre régal; ils baillent en la regardant, ils ont assez de sa grâce et de sa beauté. Mais une femme qui

est un homme, une robe de la bonne faiseuse, dans laquelle est enfermé un grand gaillard barbu, voilà qui jette l'esprit dans des curiosités piquantes, voilà qui est excellent pour secouer l'ennui rassasié et faire reprendre goût à l'existence.][11]

In both articles Zola evokes the fall of the Roman empire as a model for that of the Second Empire. Georges Saint-Paul, a doctor friend of his to whom Zola had sent the autobiography, or confession, he had received from a young Italian homosexual ("Novel of a Born Invert"), describes Zola's feelings on a subject he carefully avoided in his novels:

> The sight of and especially the contact with inverts were unpleasant to Zola. "I met some on social occasions," he told me one day, "and shaking their hands gives me an instinctual feeling of repulsion, a feeling that is hard for me to control." . . . He told me one day: "How many seeds lost in one Parisian night—what a pity they won't produce human lives."
>
> [La vue et surtout le contact des invertis étaient désagréables à Zola. "J'en ai rencontré dans le monde, me dit-il un jour, et j'éprouve à leur serrer la main une répulsion instinctive que j'ai quelques peines à dominer." . . . Il me disait un jour: "Que de semence perdue en une nuit de Paris—quel dommage que tout cela ne donne pas des humanités."][12]

For Zola, homosexuality was emblematic of all nonreproductive sexuality, just as, in medical texts, it was the structuring figure in a rhetoric medicalizing sexuality. In Zola's rhetoric, it is an antisocial, antinational activity. Its sterility was one of its most alarming aspects at a time of generalized birthrate paranoia in France. Sterility was also the sign that one had reached the final stages of degeneration. Zola, however, never directly dealt with the "problem" of male homosexuality, as he did with alcoholism or prostitution. Too risky, probably, when he was trying to be elected to the Académie Française. Yet Zola was no stranger to scandal and controversy, and his involvement in the Dreyfus affair actually required far more courage. So why this reluctance?

In fact, Zola's preparatory notes for *La curée* (the second novel in the Rougon-Macquart cycle), as well as the earlier versions of that novel, show that he intended to deal more frankly with the issue through the character of Maxime, an effeminate young pervert he refers to as a *petit crevé*. In his notes, he describes Maxime as "one of those runts, robustly named '*petits crevés*'" ["un de ces avortons, que l'on nomme avec énergie 'des petits crevés'" (*Les Rougon-Macquart,* vol. 5, 1772)]. Zola's rhetorical choice, here, is particularly telling. The act of naming robustly is twice performative: it constructs what it names, but also, in the same gesture, it constructs the one who names as the virile, robust opposite of the effeminate man. As John Lapp observes, "True to his program, Zola had desired to portray effeminacy, not for its own sake, but as the dramatic proof of a blemished heredity."[13] Yet, he would not deal as directly with the topic of male homosexuality as he did with female homosexuality in *Nana*. According to Lapp, "Traditional tolerance of Lesbianism . . . made it possible for him to introduce the Sapphic episodes in *Nana;* male inversion was out of the question" (283). Was it, as Lapp suggests, Zola's correspondence with the homosexual author of the "Novel of a Born Invert" which made him realize that some perverts actually suffered from their vices, thus making it difficult for him to use male homosexuality as a literary device?

The answer may have something to do with the fact that Zola never quite manages to fetishize completely the figure of the homosexual so as to make it signify in a heterotextual system of meaning. For his friend Dr. Georges Saint-Paul, writing under the name of Laupts, the task of the sexologist is the following:

To study the use of the malformed and the unfortunate, of the impotent, the inverts, the unhappy and unfit for marriage, the desperate, drifting toward suicide . . . in a word of those who constitute today a *true social waste*. . . . I hope someday to devote a book to the question of *the use of social waste* in future societies. (original emphasis)

[Etudier l'utilisation des malformés et des malchanceux, impuissants, invertis, malheureux et inaptes au mariage, désespérés évoluant vers le suicide . . . en un mot de ceux qui constituent à l'heure actuelle *un véritable déchet social*. . . . J'espère pouvoir consacrer ultérieurement un ouvrage à l'importante question de *l'utilisation des déchets sociaux* dans les sociétés de l'avenir. (Laupts [Saint-Paul], *L'homosexualité et les types homosexuels*, 385; original emphasis)]

But Zola never manages to sever the social link radically and make the homosexual the significant reject of the greater bourgeois narrative.

In *La débâcle,* two characters are implicitly constructed in terms of homosexuality: the emperor Napoleon III and Maurice, who is one of the two protagonists of the novel. In both cases, Zola is unable to hide the affection he feels for these characters. But while the former clearly represents a clinical case of degeneracy, the latter, in his relation to Jean, the other protagonist, better reveals Zola's hesitation and the disruption of his initial project.

Queering Napoleon III?

La débâcle is not the first novel in the cycle in which Napoleon III appears. In *Son excellence Eugène Rougon* and *L'argent*, Zola had already described the emperor as a sensualist and made him the symbol of the sexual decadence of the Second Empire. In *La débâcle*, following a narrative technique modeled on the medical discourse of Zola's period, which considers the individual as a symbol for the group, the physical decline of Napoleon III mirrors the breakdown of the regime and the nation. To be sure, Zola was not the only one in France to place the blame for the defeat against Prussia on a corrupt regime, headed by a depraved, gambling emperor, as if the catastrophe of 1870 had been the price to pay for the sins of the empire.[14] Zola describes the downfall of the regime as "the collapse of their whole world, the Second Empire swept away in the swirling torrent of its vices and mistakes" (394) ["l'effondrement d'un monde, le second Empire emporté dans la débâcle de ses vices et de ses fautes" (801)], and the Paris Commune that followed it as the result "of the evil ferments of the previous reign" (my translation) ["des ferments mauvais du dernier règne" (871)]. Throughout the novel, the regular appearances of an increasingly pathetic Napoleon, suffering from chronic diarrhea, emptying himself of his excrements, symbolically punctuate the stages of the French defeat. As in the case of Mac-Mahon's wounded buttocks, the cause of the empire's downfall seems to be located somewhere around the rectal area of its leaders.

Zola's portrait of the emperor, beyond the possible symbolism of diarrhea as a call for a great national purge, directly echoes the clinical descriptions of the abulic: fatalistic, indecisive, yet subject to sudden outbursts of irrational activity: "a conspirator, a dreamer whose energy fails him when the moment for action arrives" (60) ["C'était le conspirateur, le rêveur à qui l'énergie manque au moment de l'action" (458–59)]. The collapse of his will soon entails the loss of his identity, and the emperor is no more than "the shadowy figure [who] came and went, resigned to the inevitability of the sacrifice" (100) ["l'ombre [qui] allait et revenait sans cesse, résignée à la fatalité du sacrifice" (499)]; "he had remained in the background . . . resigned to being nothing but a nameless, tiresome nonentity, a troublesome package" (269) ["il s'était effacé . . . résigné à n'être qu'une inutilité sans nom et encombrante" (669)]. As the novel progresses, his complexion becomes more and more livid. But it is especially in his gaze that his downfall, and that of France, can be seen.

The gaze constitutes, for Zola, the main instrument by which to acquire knowledge, that is, power. When the emperor first appears in the novel, Doctor

Bouroche, who represents everything a man of science should be, takes one look and makes his diagnosis: "Done for!" (60) ["Foutu!" (458)]. The degradation or fragmentation of the gaze, however, figures the absence of global comprehension and the loss of power. Napoleon's destiny is entirely contained in his eyes, Zola insists. He describes his "dim, wavering, watery eyes" (60) ["les yeux vacillants, comme troubles et pleins d'eau" (458)]; and later, he repeats these adjectives: "those same dim, wavering, watery eyes which had characterized his appearance in Rheims" (97) ["ces yeux vacillants, troubles et pleins d'eau, qu'il avait déjà à Reims" (495–96)]. The emperor is said to have "gloomy eyes" (154) ["son oeil morne" (550)]; "eyes grown dim" (167) ["les yeux éteints" (563)], or "bleary eyes" (183) ["aux yeux troubles" (579)]; finally: "beneath their heavy lids the lifeless eyes expressed the resignation of a man who had gambled against fate and lost the final throw" (268) ["l'oeil mort, voilé des paupières lourdes, disait la résignation du fataliste qui avait joué et perdu contre le destin la partie dernière" (668)]. In contrast, King William of Prussia dominates the battlefield from his command post atop a hill. His gaze provides him with a global understanding of the events and the power to influence their outcome.[15] King William has the same masculine gaze as Doctor Bouroche, the surgeon, or as Zola, the experimental novelist—unlike Napoleon, who lacks the faculty to reason and synthesize which supposedly characterizes masculine intelligence.

Napoleon III becomes increasingly feminized. As I mentioned earlier, in the discourse of dégénérescence, vice leads to all vices, and in particular to homosexuality, which signifies them all. A depraved man, even a heterosexual man such as the emperor, is always a potential homosexual. Remember Zola's own comments on the empire's orgies. Losing control of one's will, giving in to appetites and dreams (we recall that the emperor, who has a nervous tic, is also a gambler and a smoker), suggests an effeminacy of the mind. In "Epidemics of the Will," Eve Kosofsky Sedgwick underscores the link between homosexuality and pathological addiction in nineteenth-century taxonomies. Indeed, both result from the loss of individual will. A gambler, an opium addict, an alcoholic are always predisposed to homosexuality. In Zola's novel, the succession of events portrays an increasingly symbolic feminization of the emperor, a feminization already inscribed in his degeneracy and whose early symptoms take the form of abulia or neurasthenia.

In the novel, the downfall of the Second Empire is repeatedly contrasted with the glory of the First, and once again the concept of degeneration provides a perfect explanation for an otherwise incomprehensible reversal. The generals are no longer unassuming heroes, like those of the Great Army, but a vile clique of conspirators, corrupted and softened by the pleasures of the city, a breeding ground for homosexuality. The emperor, as head of state and chief of the army, hopes to redeem the regime's vices by making the sacrifice of his life. One can read on his body the marks or symptoms of the vices he symbolically embodies, as a *pharmakos,* to protect the community. The downfall proceeds scientifically from then on. Zola, legitimated by medical discourse, can now leave his character to his inevitable degeneration, following the model he laid out in *Le roman expérimental.*

As the reality of his being progressively disappears, Napoleon, ill and powerless, can only go through the motions. Publicly, he plays the masquerade of the empire and, with his face made up like that of the aging queen of medical texts and caricatures, he reveals the deeper truth of the regime. Delaherche, one of the secondary characters in the novel, sees him as follows:

> It really was Napoleon III. He looked taller mounted on horseback and his moustaches were so heavily waxed, his cheeks so highly colored that Delaherche at once concluded that, like an actor, he had made himself up to look younger. Obviously he had had this done so that his army should not be demoralized by the sight of those cadaverous features drawn with suffering, that pinched-looking nose, those bleary eyes. And as soon as he heard that fighting had broken out at Bazeilles, he had ridden straight here, but as subdued, doleful and ghastly as ever, despite the rouge with which he had touched up his cheeks. (183)

> [C'était bien Napoléon III, qui lui apparaissait plus grand, à cheval, et les moustaches si fortement cirées, les joues si colorées, qu'il le jugea tout de suite rajeuni, fardé comme un acteur. Sûrement, il s'était fait peindre, pour ne pas promener, parmi son armée, l'effroi de son masque blême, décomposé par la souffrance, au nez aminci, aux yeux troubles. Et, averti dès cinq heures qu'on se battait à Bazeilles, il était venu, de son air silencieux et morne de fantôme, aux chairs ravivées de vermillon. (579)]

The comparison with an actor attributes a particular set of negative connotations to the emperor. The profession was at the time closely associated with homosexuality (for men, and with prostitution for women). The best-known version of this stereotypical portrait can be found in *Death in Venice,* where Thomas Mann describes in a similar fashion the pathetic end of Aschenbach. Ever since homosexuality entered medical books, its folklore seems to have been nothing more than a tragic clown show designed to hide the reality of a morbid destiny, a destiny of degeneration. Up to the end, the emperor, no longer his own master, is deprived of the heroic and redeeming death he desperately seeks:

Evidently, death had rejected him. The anxiety of his journey through defeat had made the sweat pour down his face and washed away his make up and melted his waxed moustache, while his ashen face had assumed the mournful, bewildered expression of a man on the point of death. (224)

[La mort n'avait pas voulu de lui, décidément. Sous la sueur d'angoisse de cette marche au travers de la défaite, le fard s'en été allé des joues, les moustaches cirées s'étaient amollies, pendantes, la face terreuse avait pris l'hébétement douloureux d'une agonie. (621)] [16]

The transmission of power which soon takes place, from the emperor to the empress, adds to Napoleon's feminization. From Paris, a symbol of imperial debauchery, the empress makes Bazaine the commander in chief of the armed forces and assumes power herself, reversing gender roles and symbolically stripping Napoleon of his manhood. Everything in the descriptions of the character seems to suggest a symbolic homosexualization, which allows Zola not only to stick to the theories of degeneration structuring his technique of character development, but also to link two metonymies with one metaphor: by making the emperor a metaphoric homosexual, he connects the metonymy which substitutes the emperor for the empire with the one which substitutes homosexuality for degeneration. To the empire's degeneration, then, corresponds, in the text, the emperor's homosexuality.

Such a structural role in the overall narrative can be assigned to the character precisely because of this transformation: progressively constructed as a foreign body, as Other, Napoleon can now be symbolically rejected. In a way, the character's recurring appearances represent a double process of evocation and repression, a determining aspect, as we shall see, in the relationship between Jean and Maurice. The figure of the homosexual which informs the clinical portrait of the emperor is an empty, available signifier, used to condense into one pathological type all the fears inspired by dégénérescence—yet another unstable signifier. All these fears, then, converge on the emperor. They are sometimes specific fears such as sterility or the loss of one's will; more often they are the overall fear of dégénérescence itself, that is, a concept so vague, so undefinable, but so terrifying that to symbolize it becomes the only way to keep it at a safe distance. The homosexual is a lightning rod, a role the emperor seems aware of as his repeated, and unsuccessful, attempts to get killed seem to indicate. In this sense, Zola's writing of "the homosexual" through the character of Napoleon III is a success, insofar as it fits the role assigned to it by medical discourse, and despite the fact that the author cannot hide his sympathy for this tragic character. Maurice's homosexuality, however, seems to escape Zola's control, and entails a disruption of the narration.

The Rambling Degenerate and the Instability of Authorship

Needless to say, the homosexual dimension of Maurice's character has to be decoded. In spite of the homoerotic charge of certain scenes, Zola is careful not to cross the line and present his characters in explicitly sexual terms. Yet, right from the start, Maurice's portrayal, like Napoleon's, corresponds to certain overdetermined, clinical descriptions. First of all, Maurice is a man who unsuccessfully tried to change class. Born a peasant, he moved to Paris to pursue a legal career. We know of the big city's negative connotations in Zola's work, as well as in post-Rousseauistic literature in general.[17] In addition, the idea of *déclassement* is also closely linked to clichés about homosexuality. There was a widespread perception at the time that many homosexual relationships involved rich bourgeois and especially aristocrats implicated in illicit affairs with young peasants or workingmen more or less used as kept boys. Such a perception, whether justified or not, was enough to make homosexuality the very type of sexuality that threatened the bourgeois order by destabilizing the class system the way it destabilized gender. Maurice's attempted shift from one social class to another carries with it all these connotations.

Physically and mentally, he is "almost a woman," as Zola wrote in his early notes for *La débâcle*.[18] In the novel, Maurice, not unlike the emperor, exhibits all the symptoms of abulia; he is a man with weak nerves and delicate, feminine features:

> His presence here as a volunteer was the aftermath of years of dissipation and wrongdoing resulting from a weak, impetuous nature. Oh, the money he had thrown away on gambling and on women and on all the wild pleasures of Paris, that predatory city where he had been sent to complete his studies at the expense of a family which had pinched and scraped in their efforts to make a gentleman of him. . . . Today Maurice regarded himself as thoroughly reformed; he was highly strung, full of high hopes at one moment and of dark despondency at the next; although a man of generous enthusiasms, he had no more consistency than a weathercock. He was

a short, fair-haired figure; beneath the bulging brow, the narrow face showed a small nose and chin and a pair of soft grey eyes which at times took on a somewhat crazy look. (5)

[Et, s'il se trouvait là, engagé volontaire, c'était à la suite de grandes fautes, toute une dissipation de tempérament faible et exalté, de l'argent qu'il avait jeté au jeu, aux femmes, aux sottises de Paris dévorateur, lorsqu'il y était venu terminer son droit et que la famille s'était saignée pour faire de lui un monsieur. . . . Et Maurice se croyait bien corrigé, dans sa nervosité prompte à l'espoir du bien comme au découragement du mal, généreux, enthousiaste, mais sans fixité aucune, soumis à toutes les sautes du vent qui passe. Blond, petit, avec un front très développé, un nez et un menton menus, le visage fin, il avait des yeux gris et caressants, un peu fous parfois. (405)]

The feminine connotations are easy to recognize: weak nerves, frivolity, softness, indecision, and so on. At times Zola is even more explicit: "weak and nervous as a woman, he sank into a mood of deep despair in which his whole world seemed to be foundering" (314) ["d'une faiblesse de femme, il cédait à un de ces désespoirs immenses, où le monde entier sombrait" (715)]. Maurice is constantly prey to sudden mood swings, extravagant thoughts, fevers, obsessive ideas, exaltation, and other similar symptoms. As with Napoleon, Zola uses Maurice's effeminacy to represent the degeneracy of the national community as a whole: "As highly-strung as a woman, unsettled by the sickness of the times, a victim of the historical and social crisis through which the French race was passing, as capable of rising to the noblest enthusiasm, at a moment's notice, as of sinking into the blackest depression" (162) ["D'une nervosité de femme, ébranlé par la maladie de l'époque, subissant la crise historique et sociale de la race, capable d'un instant à l'autre des enthousiasmes les plus nobles et des pires découragements" (557–58)]. Moreover, his shift in social class, from poor provincial to Parisian lawyer, entails his misplaced attraction for bad science, a partial and fragmented knowledge he is unable to use toward constructive ends. His life is a "ghost-ridden nightmare":

It was as though he were advancing towards an abyss in the full knowledge that it lay somewhere ahead, waiting to engulf him. The experience was undermining his whole outlook as an educated man; it was dragging him down to the level of the wretches who surrounded him. (28)

[Il n'avançait plus que dans un cauchemar d'atroce lassitude, halluciné de fantômes, comme s'il allait à un gouffre, là-bas, devant lui; et c'était une dépression de toute sa culture d'homme instruit, un abaissement qui le tirait à la bassesse des misérables dont il était entouré. (427)]

Again, what we read here is the bourgeois narrative of *dégénérescence,* in which the individual who separates himself from his "natural" class and gender enters into an unrelenting process of regression. Later, Maurice is "swayed by his reading again" (164) ["repris par sa science" (560)]: "Once again he was caught in the trap of self-delusion. He was so highly strung that he needed continual self-deception" (165) ["De nouveau, l'illusion vivace le tenait, tout un besoin d'aveuglement, dans l'exagération maladive de sa sensibilité nerveuse" (560)]. For Zola, science in the wrong hands can only lead to degeneracy and self-destruction. Maurice, for instance, was "analyzing himself with an ever more acute awareness of his own defects" (313) [Maurice "raisonnait le mal, s'analysant, retrouvant aiguisée la faculté de se dévorer lui-même" (715)]. He is just lucid enough to realize that his own downfall is inextricably linked to that of the nation:

> And this degeneration of the race, which seemed to explain how France, victorious only two generations ago, had now been defeated, weighed upon his mind like some hereditary disease, which, slowly getting worse, leads to inevitable destruction when the hour strikes. (313–14)

> [Et cette dégénérescence de la race, qui expliquait comment la France victorieuse avec les grands-pères avait pu être battue dans les petits-fils, lui écrasait le coeur, telle qu'une maladie de famille, lentement aggravée, aboutissant à la destruction fatale, quand l'heure avait sonné. (715)]

Already too affected himself, he is unable to do anything about his own fate.

The social and sexual ambivalence of Maurice, perceived as pathological, is represented in the text as a division of his personality: "His misdeeds in Paris had never been anything but acts of madness committed by what he termed his 'other self,' by the weakling he turned into at moments of desperation, a creature capable of the vilest conduct" (26) ["Ses fautes, à Paris, n'avaient jamais été que les folies de 'l'autre,' comme il disait, du garçon faible qu'il devenait aux heures lâches, capable des pires vilenies" (425)]. What we read here is the Jekyll-and-Hyde structure of *dégénérescence* as the malevolent reverse of positive progress, as the Same becoming Other. In addition, Maurice has a twin sister, Henriette, thanks to whom Zola can physically separate Maurice's feminine Other and resolve, through a narrative artifice, the dilemma of his relationship with Jean.

Maurice's relationship with Jean, although never explicitly sexual, does have an undeniable homoerotic component. It is interesting for a lot of different reasons to notice that this dimension has been systematically neglected by nearly all Zola scholars. Michel Serres, for instance, sees only a fraternal relationship, or a father/son relationship, which is not altogether untrue, but he somehow refuses to step out of the heterosexual model to explain the Same/Other relationship which constitutes the basis of his analysis of *La débâcle*. What is unspoken in the novel remains so in critical writings. Naomi Schor seems to be the only one to have proposed a serious, although incomplete, study of the homosexual aspects of Jean and Maurice.[19] I will come back to this later.

The relationship between the two characters starts with mutual contempt between the city and the country, which they represent. Each symbolizing one half of a divided France, the return to national harmony depends on that of the characters. Soon, their friendship is sealed by an exchange of cigarettes, and from this moment on, Zola describes Jean, the country boy, in feminine terms also; it is, however, as a nurturing, motherly figure and not as that of the hysteric urban woman used in portraying Maurice. When taking care of Maurice, Jean's "actions were almost motherly: into them went all the gentleness of a man of experience whose thick fingers were capable of extreme delicacy when the occasion arose" (83) ["il avait des gestes maternels, toute une douceur d'homme expérimenté, dont les gros doigts savent être délicats à l'occasion" (481)]. Later, Maurice realizes: "Never had the touch of a woman's arm brought such warmth to his heart" (124) ["Jamais bras de femme ne lui avait tenu aussi chaud au coeur" (521)]. Jean places Maurice in the position left vacant by the death of his wife:

> Since the violent death of his wife, carried off in circumstances of appalling tragedy, he had imagined that his heart was closed forever: he had vowed that he would always keep away from any of those creatures who cause a man so much pain, even when there is no malice in them. And to both men, friendship was becoming a kind of enlargement: although they didn't kiss, they touched each other deeply, as if they were inside one another. (125; translation modified)

> [Depuis la mort violente de sa femme, emportée dans un affreux drame, il avait juré de ne plus en voir, de ces créatures dont on souffre tant, même quand elles ne sont pas mauvaises. Et l'amitié leur devenait à tous deux comme un élargissement: on avait beau ne pas s'embrasser, on se touchait à fond, on était l'un dans l'autre. (521)]

As the story unfolds, the two characters find themselves alone at night after their escape:

They clung together, united in the fellowship of suffering, and the kiss they exchanged seemed to them sweeter and stronger than any they had yet experienced, and the like of which they would never receive from women, a pledge of eternal friendship, given in the absolute conviction that henceforward the two of them would be as one. (379; translation modified)

[Et ils se serraient d'une étreinte éperdue, dans la fraternité de tout ce qu'ils venaient de souffrir ensemble; et le baiser qu'ils échangèrent alors parut le plus doux et le plus fort de leur vie, un baiser tel qu'ils n'en recevraient jamais d'une femme, l'immortelle amitié, l'absolue certitude que leurs deux coeurs n'en faisaient plus qu'un pour toujours. 785)]

These passages in which Zola describes the feelings Jean and Maurice have for one another precisely represent the type of exalted friendships that develop in environments (like boarding schools or the army) Zola himself criticized so emphatically because they supposedly fostered homosexuality. What is crucial here is that the homoeroticism of these scenes couldn't be further from the pathological homosexuality of the emperor. Zola seems to be saying something else here.

These love scenes—and I am using the term in the broadest possible sense—soon take on mythical accents. One can easily read Christian connotations in the passage where Jean, down on his knees, washes Maurice's wounded feet. Soon, the relationship becomes "the brotherliness which had existed in the early days of the world, the brand of friendship which had preceded all barriers of class and education" (124) ["la fraternité des premiers jours du monde, l'amitié avant toute culture et toute classe" (521)]; and later on: "The brotherhood that had grown between this peasant and himself went into the depth of his being, the root of life itself. This went back, perhaps, to the first days of the world, and it was as if there were only two men left" (my translation) ["La fraternité qui avait grandi entre ce paysan et lui, allait au fond de son être, à la racine même de la vie. Cela remontait peut-être aux premiers jours du monde, et c'était comme s'il n'y avait plus eu que deux hommes" (663)]. It is true that these passages reflect Maurice's point of view, and we know that he is prone to pathological exaggerations. Nevertheless, it is also true that they express Zola's dream of a return to the long-lost unity of the national community. In the text, this return to the founding myth of humanity may recall the Christian myth of Genesis, only with two men this time, or, more accurately perhaps, Plato's *Symposium*. The recurring reunions of Jean and Maurice directly conjure up the reunification of the two halves of one of the original beings, in this case the one who was twice male. Serres rightly describes this bond as "a brotherhood above all contract. A bond preceding language" ["une fraternité par-dessus tout contrat. Un lien précédant le langage" (320)].

Indeed, when the first kiss takes place, the narration is momentarily put on hold, and Zola's naturalistic language becomes romantic. By situating the scene not just in a natural setting but in complete darkness and silence, he tones down all the realistic details so typical of his descriptive style, as well as the narrative movement of the novel. In this scene, Zola sets aside "reality" and leaves only the movements of the heart and pure lyricism:

> Once they were in the wood, in the huge, dark silence, where nothing stirred among the motionless trees, they felt they were safe, and with a feeling of extraordinary exhilaration they threw themselves into each other's arms. Maurice was sobbing as though his heart would break, and even Jean was in tears. (379)

> [Dans le bois, dans le grand silence noir des arbres immobiles, quand ils n'entendirent plus rien, que plus rien ne remua et qu'ils se crurent sauvés, une émotion extraordinaire les jeta aux bras l'un de l'autre. Maurice pleurait à gros sanglots, tandis que des larmes lentes coulaient sur les joues de Jean. (785)]

In the French text, Zola uses the term *ruisseler,* which echoes the streams of blood in the amputation scenes.[20] In both cases, the plot seems to pause. The narration is disrupted in such scenes, which have little if any narrative purpose, and serve mainly as metaphors for the ideas developed in *Le roman expérimental:* the amputation of rotten limbs from the body politic on the one hand, and the regained harmony of the city and the country on the other. Beizer reads a symbolic feminization in the blood streams of the hospital scenes, which she likens to menstrual blood, a factor of regeneration. To this I will add that Zola homosexualizes his narration when he projects, through Jean and Maurice, a symbolic image of the ideal community of the future—precisely when one would expect heterosexuality and procreation.[21]

A scene like this one, in which Zola's style becomes romantic and "feminine," to reuse his own terms from *Le roman expérimental,* threatens the very writing of the novel and the author's project. For the narrative to take place, one must exclude homosexuality so that only a homosocial bond may remain.[22] As Schor remarks: "There is no question but that in *La débâcle,* Zola went as far as he could in depicting a male homosexual relationship. . . . Zola finds himself here at a point of no return: either he goes on to show the consummation of this love affair or else he must find some expedient to divert the characters' and the readers' attention/libido" (*Zola's Crowds*, 116–17). The expedient will be Henriette, Maurice's twin sister, onto whom Jean safely transfers his feelings, and who plays here the classic role of mediator of male homosexual desire. Her introduction in the novel is all the more artificial in that it jeopardizes the whole experiment. The basic theory of the experimental novel required that the characters be left to their natural evolution in a given environment, the novelist simply observing and recording the results. Yet, in *La débâcle,* homosexuality is at the end of what Schor calls "the natural course of events" (117). To restore order in the text, Zola *must* invent Henriette and kill Maurice.

The reason why the homosexual drift in *La débâcle* has to be interrupted is that it disrupts the scientific, naturalistic discourse. It reveals an archaic or mythical intertext which radically contradicts the initial project. I have already underscored the Platonic undertones of the homosexual relationship of Jean and Maurice. For Schor: "Homosexual love, whether consummated or not, in keeping with Platonic tradition is conceived of as a higher form of love, where devotion looms larger than selfishness, where a primitive unity is restored" (117). This relationship, then, which explicitly conjures up the origins of the world, also evokes the myth of the perfect being whose fall from grace is the structuring metaphor in the rhetoric of *dégénérescence.* Two myths of the original man intersect here and, as Zola seems to suggest unwittingly, homoeroticism appears to be the ideal way to return to the state of plenitude figured in those myths.

It is significant to notice that the character of Maurice became more important in the novel than Zola had originally planned. It was Jean who was supposed to be the central protagonist, whereas Maurice's purpose was to provide a symbolic counterexample. David Baguley analyzes in detail the structural importance as a character of Maurice, who, up to the Paris Commune episode at the end of the novel, rises above the immanence of the events almost to become a narrator. Baguley, however, falls short of considering the problems posed by this narrator's homosexuality.[23] Schor, as we have seen, does consider it, but mostly at a thematic level, as if Zola's only problem was to avoid dealing openly with the *theme* of homosexuality. When she rightly remarks that for Zola "homosexuality and revolution are metaphors for each other"—indeed they are closely linked in the bourgeois rhetoric of *dégénérescence*—she stops one step too soon, as she writes that Maurice's sacrifice "is considered necessary if the health of the body politic is to be restored" (118). By killing Maurice, Zola actually attempts to regain control over a narrative which had escaped him as soon as he had entrusted it to an unstable and fragmented narrator.

Toward the end of *La débâcle,* a dying Maurice reveals the deeper coherence both of the events and the text by applying to himself the metaphor of the rotten limb that must be amputated for the community to survive: "Well, I'm that rotten limb" (494) ["Eh bien, c'est moi qui suis le membre gâté que tu as abattu" (907)]; a metaphor Jean, too, had used earlier but "finding the words with difficulty" (314) ["péniblement, au petit bonheur des mots" (716)], not fully aware of the deep meaning of a language he has not mastered very well. In contrast, when Maurice uses the same metaphor he, as Serres writes: "becomes delirious and delivers the truth. The truth of the text by the delirious text" ["entre en délire et délivre la vérité. La vérité du texte par le texte en délire" (323)]. Zola writes:

> He was growing more and more excited. . . . With feverish energy he elaborated his theme, in a succession of symbols and striking images. It was the healthy part of France, the sensible, well-balanced peasants that had always remained close to the soil, which was now ridding the country of that other frantic, crazy element that had been ruined by the Empire, misled by its day-dreams and self-indulgence. (494)

> [Et il continuait, dans une fièvre chaude, abondante en symboles, en images éclatantes. C'était la partie saine de la France, la raisonnable, la pondérée, la paysanne, celle qui était restée le plus près de la terre, qui supprimait la partie folle, exaspérée, gâtée par l'empire, détraquée de rêveries et de jouissance. (907)]

Who is speaking here? By placing almost word for word the rhetoric of the author in the mouth of the character, the author provides for the character a certain authority (in the etymological sense of the term, but also as we say that a doctor or a text is an authority on a given subject). This authority is similar to the authority Zola confers upon himself, as if Maurice's delirium were his own. Unlike Jean, for whom a metaphor is hardly ever more than a maxim, good old peasant common sense, Maurice, like Zola, possesses a global view of the situation.[24] He understands the metaphorical nature of his relationship to Jean, that is, he treads on the author's territory. To talk about oneself not in metaphorical terms but as a metaphor is not, by definition, an attribute of the naturalistic character, a passive object moved by forces beyond his control or his understanding. Indeed, how could a textuality so entirely concerned with the *effet de réel* admit meta-discursivity? Even more troubling, considering Zola's proclaimed intentions—that is, the performativity of the novel as genre—is the fact that one would have expected Jean, the healthy carrier of hope in a future community, to be the spokesman for his theories. Originally, Jean was to represent these theories in *La débâcle*, right before the arrival of Doctor Pascal, in the following novel, who would be in charge of closing the cycle. But Zola, as we have seen, lets himself be overwhelmed by Maurice's character and ends up surrendering to him the supreme authority, his own.[25]

This narrative slippage undermines the carefully constructed image of the experimental novelist. When appropriating the image of the late-nineteenth-century doctor, Zola mainly intended to incorporate its heroic connotations. Yet, because of his identification with Maurice, that is, with the ill, the degenerate, the potential invert, Zola ceased to present himself as the omnipotent, omniscient surgeon performing wholesome amputations on the body politic. Instead, he himself became the rotten limb. He was no longer the master of a normative language constructing the Other by means of the disease metaphor. Such a displacement was made possible by the fact that the experimental novelist was unable to maintain the safe distance between the empiricist and his subject, and instead, implicated himself in the text in a subjective, delirious, self-referential, romantic fashion. Such a loss of control, accidental though it may be, is still crucial: it indicates that the figure of the experimental novelist, like that of the doctor it mimics, is actually a metaphorical construct. Just as the metaphor of *dégénérescence* both reflects and reveals the metaphor of progress, other structuring dichotomies such as healthy/pathological, heterosexual/homosexual, doctor/patient, author/character tell of a similar relation of mutual dependence between opposite signifiers. The case of Maurice, then, does not represent an anomaly in Zola's discourse; rather it reveals the meta-discursive nature of a textuality caught in a self-contained system of metaphor and self-reference. In fact, what Zola unintentionally exposes (for others to exploit) is the radical homosexualization always already contained within modernity itself as well as modernity's built-in potential for self-destruction. As we shall see in the following chapters, Jean Genet and Hervé Guibert attempt to subvert mechanisms of power by actively assuming the dual positioning Zola revealed only inadvertently.

3

℘

Reclaiming Disease and Infection

Jean Genet and the Politics of the Border

With Jean Genet's 1949 autobiographical novel, *Journal du voleur,* this study crosses over to a rhetorical "other side." Unlike Zola, Genet uses disease tropes in order to reverse them, and to write from the point of view of the foreign body. The purpose here is no longer to heal the community through the novel, but rather to infect and subvert both. *Journal du voleur,* narrated in the first person, presents itself as an autobiographical account of the somewhat mysterious period in Genet's life when he was making a living as a prostitute, beggar, and smuggler.[1] The *Journal's* narrator, a homosexual and a criminal, seems to be the perfect embodiment of the degenerate, whose figure was constructed in and by late-nineteenth-century medical discourse.[2] Specifically, Genet makes ample use of hygiene tropes, as he describes his characters as cesspools of infectious germs threatening what is usually referred to as public health, that is, the overall state of health of the nation-state.

Genet's text, then, works from within the normative framework of dominant medical discourse. Furthermore, by claiming the role of infectious agent forcibly assigned to him by that discourse, the narrator actively assumes all the implications of that role in terms of abjection, contamination, and so on. The inherent ambiguity of that position entails a series of questions: To what extent does Genet succeed in disrupting a discourse he has chosen to inhabit? Further, doesn't that strategy, somewhat akin to literary hijacking, end up reinforcing the very norms it seeks to subvert? In the previous chapters we saw the regulating power of biomedical discourse and its appropriation in literary enterprises using the novel to heal a national community rhetorically constructed as an organic body. Could that same genre cease to be an agent of healing to become one of contamination and disease? In other words: Is Jean Genet contagious? Or: Does the novelist thief, to borrow Edmund White's term,[3] have the ability to contaminate the social and symbolic order whose entire purpose is to exclude him? In order to address these questions, I approach *Journal du voleur* in three broad movements: how Genet deploys a rhetoric of leprosy and lice to arrive at a paradox—the representation of the abject; how language itself becomes object and factor of contamination and border crossing; finally how, by positioning himself at the border, Genet ultimately proposes a radical deterritorialization of the subject.[4]

Before moving on to the *Journal du voleur* itself, I need to clarify a few theoretical assumptions that I use as my starting points. In what follows, I use the terms "order" and "system" pretty much interchangeably to mean the concept of social and symbolic order in general, and not, unless otherwise indicated, a particular order or system. I define an order, or system, as a power structure founded by an act of exclusion inaugurating the notions of inside and outside, on which all other dichotomies are based. The inside is the system itself; the outside is unrepresentable by definition, since all idea of representation is produced by the system—in fact, every system is a system of representation.

In the text, Genet refers explicitly to specific orders or systems—France, Europe, bourgeois culture, Western civilization—enforced by specific institutions or discourses, such as the police, the law, the church, capitalism, gender, sexuality. Each institution or discourse produces its set of defining dichotomies; but each dichotomy thus produced—police and thieves, law and outlaw, good and evil, hetero- and homosexual—contains the whole system and the very notion of order—which is what Genet is really after. Indeed, while Genet, and therefore myself in my reading of Genet, may refer to specific power structures and their corresponding dichotomies, his ultimate goal is the destabilization of the notion of order in general.

Drawing on the dictionary definition of "dichotomy" as the "division or subdivision of a class into two mutually exclusive groups,"[5] I posit the following syllogism: all dichotomies contain the inside/outside dichotomy; the inside/outside dichotomy contains the system; therefore all dichotomies contain the system. Deconstruct one and the whole system unravels.

As Genet shows us, the outside gets represented within the system as spaces assigned (with symbolic and/or physical force) to "outsiders" who are to be removed from the system. In modern Western societies, these spaces take the form of prisons, hospitals, the private sphere, and so forth. Paradoxically, these spaces, signifying exteriority, are places of confinement; from the point of view of the system, they look as if they are (en)closed. (We'll see later on how Genet's narrator feels like an insider in Nazi Germany because he is in a country considered to be "outside" by other countries.) What it means, of course, is that there really is no outside, or rather that the outside can never be conceived or represented without being automatically reinscribed inside the system of representation. Genet's emphasis on places of confinement in his work—the prison, the penal colony, the brothel, the ship, Guiana (in *Journal du voleur*), a police station, the community of beggars in Spain, et cetera—shows us that the outside is really (produced by the) inside. Genet recuperates the discourses that construct him as an outsider to show that it is precisely *as* an (absolute) outsider that he is (always) inside. While Genet's famous motto, "J'encule le monde,"[6] implies that he is *in* the world (coming in, as it were, through the back door), his desire to be fucked (that is, the fact that he embraces his identification as a "passive" homosexual) also implies that the world is in him as well. Of course, this is logically impossible—which is why the "central" theme in *Journal du voleur* is the border. That, in a sense, is Genet's poetic challenge: to take us to the impossible moment when there is no inside/outside, and therefore no system.

One last note about the organization of my reading. In a sense, *Journal du voleur* represents somewhat of a vulgarization of Genet's previous work, or at the very least a simplification of it. Championed by the likes of Sartre and Cocteau, Genet had reached national fame at that time, and his readership was about to expand dramatically. For the first time in his literary career, he knew, as he was writing *Journal du voleur,* that his work would be published by a major mainstream publisher, Gallimard, as part of its prestigious "nrf" collection. This sudden inscription within capitalist economy and bourgeois power, which makes his work what Pierre Bourdieu would call "symbolic capital,"[7] is not necessarily a sign that Genet had "sold out." As Ross Chambers points out in *Room for Maneuver:*

> [I]t is the ongoing *readability* of texts (and works of art), their ability to transcend the context of their production, that enables them to make all the necessary concessions and compromises with the prevailing power of the moment—to make use of the existing means of publication, for instance—but to do so, so to speak, as a tactic of "survival," so that their oppositional readability can become available, at a later date and in changed historical circumstances, to a readership that is the true object of their "address." (2; original emphasis)

This being said, Genet was aware of the risks, and his typical antagonistic relationship with his readers became even more outspoken, or, let's say, explicitly problematized, in *Journal du voleur*.[8] With this new text, presented, or disguised, as an autobiography, which was his last book-length narrative piece for almost forty years, Genet took the opportunity to articulate his major tenets more clearly. In an act of willing contamination, my reading takes the same form: it moves from the figural to the literal. Ultimately structured by the idea of the border, it discusses metaphorical borders first, such as the borders between dichotomies, and ends with considerations of images of "real" national borders.

Disease, Vermin, and Abjection

To depict his miserable life in the slums of Barcelona in the 1930s, Genet relies mostly on images of diseases traditionally associated with poverty, ugliness, and lack of hygiene.[9] Filth, defilement, and all possible varieties of infestations go hand in hand with the most repulsive infections. The reader can expect to see just about anything in "that vast, filthy disorder, in a neighborhood stinking of oil, piss and shit" (*The Thief's Journal*, 25) ["dans ce vaste désordre sale, au milieu d'un quartier puant l'huile, l'urine et la merde" (*Journal du voleur*, 26)]; such as "decayed teeth, foul breath, a hand cut off, smelly feet, etc." (54) ["les dents gâtées, l'haleine fétide, la main coupée, l'odeur des pieds, etc." (57)]; and immediately after: "a hand cut off, a gouged eye, a peg leg, etc. We are fallen during the time we bear the marks of the fall" (54–55) ["la main coupée, l'oeil crevé, le pilon, etc. On est déchu durant qu'on porte les marques de la déchéance" (57)]. Beyond the accumulation of sordid details, this indicates a strategy of representation that is quite different from the more traditional style of descriptions favored by Zola. Genet's use of definite articles, as well as the final "etc." that gives the reader the theoretical possibility of continuing the list, show that Genet isn't proposing a bourgeois, realistic portrayal of the world of poverty, but is in fact referring to a series of clichés about that world—indeed, marks. If the reader is able to add to the list it is because it refers not to something real that both author and reader would have witnessed, but rather to previously read and immediately recognizable descriptions. What the reader may add by continuing the list, therefore, has nothing to do with literary creation or the mimetic transcription of reality—it is more like quoting. And the same goes for the author. Unlike Zola, Genet never claims to reproduce reality. Instead, he attempts to denaturalize his descriptions—and all descriptions—precisely by exposing them as mere quotations, always already removed from their referents. In modern French culture it is not uncommon to exclaim "C'est du Zola!" to describe the downward spiral of abject poverty, thus referring not to reality but to a previously validated discourse whose codes are shared by, and indeed form, a cultural community. With his list of clichés Genet exposes the absence of an extralinguistic referential object for "the fall." "We are fallen during the time we bear the marks of the fall," that is, we are fallen only within the boundaries of the discourse that produces the fall.

Logically, Genet selects the most obvious clichés, those with the most immediate connotations. The image of leprosy falls in that category. To use leprosy as metaphor conjures up the idea of exclusion beyond the boundaries of the community toward an abjected outside figured by the lepers' colony. But it also implies that such exclusion is signified by bodily marks. As Susan Sontag writes in *Illness as Metaphor:* "Leprosy in its heyday aroused a . . . disproportionate sense of horror. In the Middle Ages, the leper was a social text in which corruption was made visible; an exemplum, an emblem of decay" (58). While leprosy was no longer as common in Europe at the time when Genet's story takes place and when the book was published, it was still virulent as a metaphor—and it still is. Sontag reminds us, for example, that "In French, a moldering façade is still *lépreuse*" (58). And it isn't uncommon to hear someone complain about being treated "like a leper."

In *Journal du voleur,* the leprosy metaphor appears both explicitly and indirectly, through identifiable connotations. Early on in the novel Genet mentions "leprosy, to which I compare our state" (27) ["La lèpre, à quoi je compare notre état" (29)]. Why choose this particular comparison? Why this disease and not another one? First, unlike the plague, which kills rapidly those it infects, leprosy allows author and reader to focus on what Genet calls a state.[10] The body of the leper thus becomes the living signifier of difference. It embodies the Other with whom all contact must be avoided.[11] The very ugliness of the leper signifies and testifies to his otherness, and his infectiousness justifies his expulsion from the world of the healthy.[12] In French, the word *immonde* comes to mind, with its double acception of "unclean" and/therefore "not of the world." This antagonistic relationship with the world of the healthy—"your world" (9) ["votre monde" (10)], Genet tells us—is a central implication of the leprosy metaphor, and one on which Genet relies heavily to depict the daily life of the group of Barcelona beggars he belongs to:

> We sometimes slept six in a bed without sheets, and at dawn we would go begging in the markets. We would leave the Barrio Chino in a group and

scatter over the Parallelo, carrying shopping baskets, for the housewives would give us a leek or turnip rather than a coin. (18)

[Nous couchions quelquefois six sur un lit sans drap et dès l'aube nous allions mendier sur les marchés. Nous quittions en bande le Barrio Chino et sur le Parallelo nous nous égrenions, un cabas au bras, car les ménagères nous donnaient plutôt un poireau ou un navet qu'un sou. (18)]

The scene directly echoes the medieval imagery of the lepers leaving their colony to beg in the marketplace.[13] But the relationship between the healthy and the sick is more ambiguous than it seems, inasmuch as it doesn't signify a radical and definitive exclusion.

In *Purity and Danger*, Mary Douglas shows that from an anthropological perspective, dirt and defilement are signs of disorder, and charity gives form to a ritualized contact with the Other. In this structure, the gift occupies more or less the same function as the sacrifice or the offering in some religious rites. The goal is to protect the community and not to establish a real communication. In fact, the begging ritual represented in Genet's text is repeated every market day and figures the reiteration of the act of exclusion performed by the gift of food. Each time, the excluded remind the community of their existence, and each time, the community has to expel them anew. The constant reminder of a kind of unwholesome, parallel world (*immonde*) simultaneously reinforces and weakens the "healthy" community it surrounds. On the one hand, it underscores and confirms *a contrario* the health of the community. On the other, it indicates that the (metaphorical) lepers' colony represents the community's constitutive boundary, and that beyond that boundary the law inverts itself.

The reader familiar with Genet's work will immediately recognize one of the bases of his poetics. To be sure, Genet does in *Journal du voleur* what he had been doing since his earliest work: he gives a positive value to what had been constructed negatively by the process of exclusion.[14] In this text, he does it (also) with the leprosy metaphor: "It is said that leprosy, to which I compare our state, causes an irritation of the tissues; the sick person scratches himself; he gets an erection. In a solitary eroticism leprosy consoles itself and hymns its disease. Poverty erected us" (27; translation modified) ["La lèpre, à quoi je compare notre état, provoquerait, dit-on, une irritation des tissus, le malade se gratte: il bande. Dans un érotisme solitaire la lèpre se console et chante son mal. La misère nous érigeait" (29)]. Erection, in this passage, is to be understood as the mirror opposite of the fall mentioned earlier. Beyond its sexual acception, the term also means the erection of a monument—that is, an official and collective recognition; in this case a monument to the glory of poverty and disease.

The specular structure that automatically comes out of the rhetorical process of inversion raises the question of the gaze, whose central role in the construction of normative health/disease dichotomies was addressed in the previous chapters. In *Journal du voleur,* we see the same gaze operating when Genet describes how a group of French tourists observe and take photographs of Barcelona's beggars. In the text, the tourists become in effect the normalizing agent that constructs the beggars' otherness. The technical terminology they use may be at times that of art criticism or ethnography or even zoology; their discourse is always one of power and exclusion. As Genet writes,

> Without considering that they might be wounding the beggars, they carried on, above their heads, an audible dialogue, the terms of which were exact and rigorous, almost technical.
>
> "There's a perfect harmony between the tonalities of the sky and the slightly greenish shades of their rags."
>
> " . . . something out of Goya . . . "
>
> "It's very interesting to watch the group on the left. There are things of Gustave Doré in which the composition . . . "
>
> "They're happier than we are."
>
> "There's something more sordid about them than those in the shantytown, you remember, in Casablanca? There's no denying that the Moroccan costume gives a *simple* beggar a dignity that no European can ever have."
>
> "We're seeing them when they're all frozen. They have to be seen when the weather is right."
>
> "On the contrary, the originality of the poses . . . " (164–65; original emphasis)

[Sans souci de les blesser, ils tinrent au dessus des mendiants un dialogue précis, dont les termes étaient nets, presque techniques.

— L'accord est parfait entre la tonalité des ciels et les teintes un peu verdâtres des loques.

— . . . ce côté Goya . . .

— Le groupe de gauche est très curieux à observer. Il y a des scènes de Gustave Doré dont la composition . . .

— Ils sont plus heureux que nous.

— Ils ont un côté plus sordide que ceux de Bidonville, vous vous souvenez, à Casa? Il faut dire que le vêtement marocain donne à un *simple* mendiant une dignité qu'un Européen ne possédera jamais.

— Nous les trouvons en plein engourdissement. Il faudrait les voir par beau temps.

— Au contraire, l'originalité des poses . . . (173–74; original emphasis)]

The tourists' discourse of authority, whether academic or scientific in its style, constructs the beggars as objects of knowledge. Just like biomedical discourse, it constructs and naturalizes the otherness of what it claims merely to describe. When the tourists take pictures of the beggars, making them artificially compose a realistic scene, it is, in fact, to reiterate the act of exclusion and to maintain a safe distance between self and other. They photograph only scenes that are reconstructed so as to correspond to a previously conceived, normalized reality:

> Like the others, Lucien stood up, leaned on his elbow, squatted, depending on the scenes the tourists wanted to immortalize. He even smiled, as ordered, at an old beggar, and he even allowed them to muss his dirty hair and make it fall down over his wet forehead. (165; translation modified)

> [Comme les autres, Lucien se mit debout, s'accouda, s'accroupit, selon les scènes que voulaient fixer les touristes. Il sourit même, comme on le lui commandait, à un vieux mendiant, et il supporta qu'on emmêlât et qu'on les rabattît sur son front mouillé ses cheveux sales. (174–75)]

As the word *fixer* indicates, the taking of photographs is used, just as it was in late-nineteenth-century medicine, to enforce the otherness of the sick while claiming to document it.

While the leprosy metaphor allows Genet to expose the mechanics of othering and to reclaim his forced identification as pathological Other, the figure of the louse helps him to radicalize his position. Just like leprosy, the louse is loaded with connotations. But whereas the disease has visible symptoms and is linked with the gaze as a reifying factor, the louse can remain mostly invisible if a proper distance is maintained. Like the rat, it is feared even when not seen, it is associated with the unhealthy, it is infectious, and it spreads epidemics. More efficiently perhaps than with the leprosy metaphor, Genet plays on the notion of hidden, lurking danger, and suggests the idea of contamination, that is, of the porosity of the boundary between the healthy world and its unclean outside, between *monde* and *immonde*. Indeed, the louse is a parasite; it lives off the vital substance of its host, the weakening of the latter insuring the strengthening of the former. But in the world of the Barrio Chino the relationship between lice and their hosts is not so stable.

Lice are everywhere in the neighborhood: "The Barrio Chino was, at the time a kind of haunt thronged less with Spaniards than with foreigners, all of them verminous bums" (25; translation modified) ["Le Barrio Chino était alors une sorte de repère peuplé moins d'Espagnols que d'étrangers qui tous étaient des voyoux pouilleux" (25)]. Lice have in fact an intimate relationship with their hosts, and Genet calls them "les poux, nos familiers" (27). And he goes on to describe the relationship of ambiguous hospitality and complicity he and his lover Salvador have with their lice:

> The lice inhabited us. They imparted to our clothes an animation, a presence, which, when they had gone, left our garments lifeless. We liked to know—and feel—that the translucent bugs were swarming; though not tamed, they were so much a part of us that a third person's louse disgusted us. We chased them away but with the hope that during the day the nits would have hatched. We crushed them with our nails, without disgust and without hatred. We did not throw their corpses—or remains—into the garbage; we let them fall, bleeding with our blood, into our untidy underclothes. (26)

> [Les poux nous habitaient. A nos vêtements ils donnaient une animation, une présence qui, disparues, font qu'ils sont morts. Nous aimions savoir—et sentir—pulluler les bêtes translucides qui, sans êtres apprivoisées, étaient si bien à nous que le pou d'un autre que de nous deux nous dégoûtait. Nous les chassions mais avec l'espoir que dans la journée les lentes auraient éclos. Avec nos ongles nous les écrasions sans dégoût et sans haine. Nous n'en jetions pas le cadavre—ou dépouille—à la voirie, nous le laissions choir, sanglant de notre sang, dans notre linge débraillé. (27)]

Genet's emphasis on the fact that the lice are bleeding with their hosts' blood indicates an identity between the two (I will come back to the radical implications of such metomymic displacement in the novel).

We can also notice that, just as he did with the leprosy metaphor, Genet uses the figure of the louse indirectly as well. For example, he mentions the fantasmatic fear of gangs of robbers who, in the chaos following World War II, were rumored to roam through the French countryside to prey upon the population: "The country was said to have been infested with them" (98) ["Le pays, a-t-on dit de la France, en était infesté" (104)]. Although implicit, the figure of the louse is conjured up by the word "infested," but also by the idea of rumors, which, just like lice, can spread as would an epidemic.[15] Once again, Genet gives a positive value to something that has been constructed in negative terms by dominant normative discourses, and lice become the emblem of a social bond, the signs of collective identification for the community they create. Indeed, for Genet, lice are tightly bound to the idea of community. But while the leprosy metaphor suggests the notion of an easily identifiable and segregated Other, the figure of the louse more effectively foregrounds the danger of contamination.

Genet describes a card game in which Stilitano, his one-armed pimp, participates:

> As I was about to take my seat, I saw a louse on the collar of his jacket. Stilitano was handsome and strong, and welcome at a gathering of similar males whose authority likewise lay in their muscles and their awareness of their revolvers. The louse on Stilitano's collar, still invisible to the other men, was not a small stray spot; it was moving; it shifted about with disturbing velocity, as if crossing and measuring its domain—its space rather. But it was not only at home; on Stilitano's collar *it was the sign that he belonged to an unmistakably verminous world,* despite his eau de Cologne and silk shirt. (61; my emphasis)

> [En me penchant pour m'asseoir, sur le col de son veston, je vis un pou. Stilitano était beau, fort, et admis dans une réunion de mâles pareils, dont l'autorité résidait également dans les muscles et dans la connaissance qu'ils avaient de leur revolver. Sur le col de Stilitano, encore invisible des autres hommes, le pou n'était pas une petite tache égarée, il se mouvait, il se déplaçait avec une vélocité inquiétante, comme s'il eût parcouru, mesuré son domaine—son espace plutôt. Mais il n'était pas seulement chez lui, sur ce col il *était le signe que Stilitano appartenait à un monde décidément pouilleux* malgré l'eau de Cologne et la chemise en soie. (64; my emphasis)]

With the idea of collective identification signified by the louse, Genet moves toward what he calls "moral abjection" ["l'abjection morale"] through "that which must be its sign: my lice, rags and filth" (59) ["ce qui doit en être le signe: mes poux, mes haillons et ma crasse" (62)]. Hence, the parasite is more than merely the thief's attribute; it becomes his emblem.

This sort of metonymic displacement is not unusual in dominant constructions of diseases, particularly of contagious and infectious diseases: given that the infectious agent—parasite, virus, bacteria—is often invisible without a microscope, it is the carrier, or anyone identified as such, who becomes the embodiment of the agent and the object of exclusion.[16] A person who carries lice becomes a louse. The panic generated by the invisibility and mobility of the infectious agent is thus alleviated by a rhetorical trick. If the purpose of the metonymy is to ensure the safety of the healthy body and its exclusionary power, it appears far more radical and effective to expel the sick than to heal them. Or rather: healing and prevention may eventually take the form of murder, or even genocide, thus exposing the inherent brutality of the metonymy. Think of the systematic construction of Jews as vermin in Nazi anti-Semitic rhetoric. Theoretically, a person carrying lice could always be deloused and rejoin the community of the healthy to which he/she had never really ceased to belong. But what can be done with the louse? And the carrier metonymically identified as a louse? Among other things, *Journal du voleur* tells us how systematic exclusion is fundamentally similar to delousing.

Yet, as I mentioned at the beginning of this chapter, Genet occupies a position within normative medical discourse. He therefore reclaims that traditional metonymic displacement and the identity it produces. But in the novel, the narrator actively assumes the process and, by doing so, disrupts his normalization as a passive victim of infection and degeneracy to become instead an active agent. The infested body is now the body politic. In the following passage, for instance, Spain is depicted as an infested space where beggars look for hospitable places just as parasites do on the body: "1932. Spain at the time was covered with vermin, its beggars. They went from village to village, to Andalusia because it is warm, to Catalonia because it is rich, but the whole country was favorable to us. I was thus a louse, and conscious of being one" (18) ["1932. L'Espagne était alors couverte de vermine, ses mendiants. Ils allaient de village en village, en Andalousie parce qu'elle est chaude, en Catalogne parce qu'elle est riche, mais tout le pays nous était favorable. Je fus donc un pou avec la conscience de l'être" (18)]. And when he adds: "It is the life of vermin that I am going to describe" (18) ["C'est les moeurs de la vermine que je vais décrire" (18)], it is clear that these descriptions will be "autobiographical"—so to speak, since Genet was a liar—and not the result of empirical observation.[17]

The first consequence of this reversal of narrative origin is the inversion of values. In a story told from the point of view of the self-proclaimed infectious agent, what had been defined as negative by biomedical discourses now becomes positive, and vice versa. The louse's value is thus reversed:

The lice were the only sign of our prosperity, of the very underside of prosperity, but it was logical that by making our state perform an operation which justified it, we were, by the same token, justifying the sign of this state. Having become as useful for the knowledge of our decline as jewels for the knowledge of what is called triumph, the lice were precious. They were both our shame and our glory. (27)

[Les poux étaient le seul signe de notre prospérité, de l'envers de la prospérité, mais il était logique qu'en faisant à notre état opérer un rétablissement qui le justifiât, nous justifiions du même coup le signe de cet état. Devenus aussi utiles pour la connaissance de notre amenuisement que les bijoux pour la connaissance de ce qu'on nomme le triomphe, les poux étaient précieux. Nous en avions à la fois honte et gloire. (27)]

From a point of view that glorifies the narrator's miserable condition, a point of view from which posterity and everything else are the opposite of what they are supposed to be in the "normal" world, lice are the equivalent of jewels. Once again, we see the disruptive specular structure so typical of Genet's work.[18] He largely reuses the type of rhetoric discussed in the first two chapters, and reverses it.

But is that all there is? A simple inversion within the same discursive model? If that were the case Genet would just be reproducing the normative discourse he inhabits without altering it. How does the "I" of "I was thus a louse" disrupt or, on the contrary, reinforce the power structure that excludes him? In *Bodies That Matter,* Judith Butler provides ways to answer these questions. From the outset she posits that the articulation of a subject position, even a resistant one, can only take place within a normative discourse: "The paradox of subjectivation (*assujettissement*) is precisely that the subject who would resist such norms is itself enabled, if not produced, by such norms. Although this constitutive constraint does not foreclose the possibility of agency, it does locate agency as a reiterative or rearticulatory practice, immanent to power, and not a relation of external opposition to power" (15). Genet was a proponent of what was known in *soixante-huitard* parlance as *entrisme*,[19] a strategy of infiltration and destruction of the system from within. He admitted the impossibility of opposing the system from the outside.[20] In *Jean Genet: Entre mythe et réalité,* Véronique Bergen rightly observes that strategic position in Genet's work. She notes:

The contradiction met by a total criticism, exempt from any inscription within the contested space, the impossibility of expressing madness by skipping over the territory of reason, of expressing the other, the different, the margin, the doomed element, Genet short-circuits all this by practicing a destabilization of order from within that order.

[La contradiction que rencontre une critique totale, exemptée de toute inscription au sein de l'espace contesté, l'impossibilité de dire la folie en sautant par-delà le territoire de la raison, de dire l'autre, le différent, la marge, la part maudite, Genet la court-circuite par sa pratique d'une déstabilisation de l'ordre menée au sein de ce dernier. (39)]

For Jonathan Dollimore, in *Sexual Dissidence,* "Genet reinscribes himself within the violent hierarchies of his oppression, installing himself there relentlessly to invert and pervert them" (314). More recently, in his preface to the special issue of *Yale French Studies* aptly entitled "Genet: In the Language of the Enemy," Scott Durham points out that Genet's work presupposes "that literary language exists in immanent relation to a discursive, libidinal, or historical outside that can be made to pass into its interior, corrupting it even in its purest forms and most elevated purposes" (3). There always remains, however, the theoretical possibility of recuperation of the subversive act by the very system one attempts to subvert. The challenge facing the subject trying to disrupt the normative discourse that enabled it is to avoid its own reconstitution as a hegemonic subject. In the absence of a miracle formula, one can still propose the following: that the agent of disruption cannot reconstitute itself as a hegemonic subject as long as it acknowledges, within itself, the absence of its constitutive outside. Which brings us to the abject.[21]

The *Journal*'s narrator often describes himself as "abject," a term that, for him, best summarizes all the reasons for his social exclusion: his poverty, his homosexuality, and his various crimes. But he adds: "Murder is not the most effective way of reaching the subterranean world of abjection" (107) ["L'assassinat n'est pas le moyen le plus efficace de rejoindre le monde souterrain de l'abjection" (113)]. For him, the most abject of crimes are the ones that are met with contempt and revulsion, which is not necessarily the result in the case of murder: "Other crimes are more degrading: theft, begging, treason, breach of trust, etc.; those are the ones I chose to commit, though I was always haunted by the idea of a murder which would cut me off irremediably from your world" (107) ["D'autres crimes sont plus avilissants: le vol, la mendicité, la trahison, l'abus de confiance, etc., c'est ceux-là que j'ai choisi de commettre, cependant que toujours je demeurais hanté par l'idée d'un meurtre qui, irrémédiablement, me retrancherait de votre monde" (113)]. What is the difference, then? Murder, the narrator specifies, would signify, in dramatic fashion, the successful exclusion of the criminal. The act of abjection that ushers in the social and symbolic order, that creates an inside and an outside, would find itself confirmed with the exclusion, and even the execution, of the murderer. But in that case, the founding act of abjection would be a ghost that haunted him. In contrast, the cunning duplicity characterizing the crimes most favored by the narrator suggests a more ambiguous type of activity. Betrayal and breach of trust, clearly his favorites, require a reappropriation and hijacking of language. Durham rightly observes that Genet's purpose is "less a matter of creating a literature of theft than of perpetrating a theft of literature; less a matter of representing a marginal subjectivity in the language of official culture than of making a subaltern or perverse use of that language itself" (2). Not unlike lies, Genet's favorite misdeeds mimic language to subvert it and to remain undetected.[22]

As Kristeva writes in *Powers of Horror:* "Any crime, because it draws attention to the fragility of the law, is abject, but premeditated crime, cunning murder, hypocritical revenge are even more so because they heighten the display of such fragility" (4) ["Tout crime, parce qu'il signale la fragilité de la loi, est abject, mais le crime prémédité, le meurtre sournois, la vengeance hypocrite le sont plus encore parce qu'ils redoublent cette exhibition de la fragilité légale" (12)]. Or in Genet's words: "I was talking about abject betrayal. The kind that cannot be justified by any heroic excuse. The sneaky, cringing kind, elicited by the least noble of sentiments: envy, hatred . . . greed" (242; translation modified) ["Je parlais de la trahison abjecte. Celle que ne justifiera aucune héroïque excuse. Celle qui est sourde, rampante, provoquée par les sentiments les moins nobles: l'envie, la haine . . . la cupidité" (257–58)].

Let's note that when Kristeva talks about "cunning murder," she does not mean the same thing as when Genet talks about murder. For Genet, as we have just seen, the murderer is precisely not abject because his action is so radical that he becomes the object of admiration (or of Genet's desire): "for he is assumed to possess, in view of the ways he defies the laws of life, the most easily imagined attributes of exceptional strength" and that "prevent[s] people from despising the criminal" (107) ["car on lui suppose, pour si bien s'opposer aux lois de la vie, les attributs les plus facilement imaginés de la force la plus grande" ce qui "empêche[] qu'on méprise ce criminel" (113)]. For Kristeva: "He who denies morality is not abject; there can be grandeur in amorality and even in crime that flaunts its disrespect for the law. . . . Abjection, on the other hand, is immoral, sinister, scheming, and shady" (4) ["Celui qui refuse la morale n'est pas abject— il peut y avoir de la grandeur dans l'amorale et même dans un crime qui affiche son irrespect de la loi. . . . L'abjection, elle, est immorale, ténébreuse, louvoyante, louche" (12)]. Therefore, for the narrator to think of himself as abject, he needs to threaten the boundary of the system. When he speaks of "reaching the subterranean world of abjection," he has not been "cut off" from the social and symbolic order, for if he had he would not be abject. Rather, he must be the embodiment of duplicity, or what Kristeva calls "[t]he in-between, the ambiguous, the composite" (4) ["L'entre-deux, l'ambigu, le mixte" (12)].

One episode, in particular, illustrates how Genet uses his idea of abjection as a threat to the system. One night, the narrator is arrested during a raid on prostitutes and their clients. At the station, his pockets are emptied, and the police find a tube of Vaseline on him:

> It concerned a tube a vaseline, one of whose ends was partially rolled up. Which amounts to saying that it had been put to use. Amidst the elegant objects taken from the pockets of the men who had been picked up in the raid, it was the sign of abjection itself, of the kind which is concealed with the greatest of care, but yet the sign of a secret grace which was soon to save me from contempt. (19–20; translation modified)

> [Il s'agissait d'un tube de vaseline dont l'une des extrémités était plusieurs fois retournée. C'est dire qu'il avait servi. Au milieu des objets élégants retirés de la poche des hommes pris dans cette rafle, il était le signe de l'abjection même, de celle qui se dissimule avec le plus grand soin, mais le signe encore d'une grâce secrète qui allait bientôt me sauver du mépris. (20)]

As the tube of Vaseline is exposed for all to see, the narrator adds:

> I was sure that this puny and most humble object would hold its own against them; by its mere presence it would be able to upset all the police in the world; it would draw down upon itself contempt, hatred, white and dumb rages. (22; translation modified)

> [j'étais sûr que ce chétif objet si humble leur tiendrait tête, par sa seule présence il saurait mettre dans tous ses états toute la police du monde, il attirerait sur soi les mépris, les haines, les rages blanches et muettes. (23)]

Using a metonymic displacement similar to the one making the carrier of lice a louse himself, Genet thus attributes his narrator's qualities to his tube of Vaseline.

What would "upset all the police in the world" is of course the purpose of the Vaseline. By searching the narrator, the policemen have themselves introduced the sign of the most abject of all sex acts, anal sex, back into the system they are supposed to symbolize and protect. Genet insists on the role of the tube of Vaseline: "that dirty, wretched object whose purpose seemed to the world—to that

concentrated delegation of the world which is the police . . . —utterly vile, became extremely precious to me" (20) ["ce misérable objet sale, dont la destination paraissait au monde—à cette délégation concentrée du monde qu'est la police . . . —des plus viles, me devint extrêmement précieux" (20–21)]; and a little
later, he mentions again "[t]he tube of vaseline whose purpose is rather well
known to you" (21; translation modified) ["Le tube de vaseline, dont la destination vous est assez connue" (22)]. In both instances, the purpose of the Vaseline
is not directly mentioned. Instead, it is defined negatively in terms of its opposition to the world, to the police, and to the readers. And because we the readers are placed in the same position as the police by Genet's use of a similar expression ("dont la destination"), it is expected that the appearance of the tube of
Vaseline in the text will produce the same destabilizing effects it produces in the
police station.

For Deleuze and Guattari, in L'anti-Oedipe, the privatization of the anus is inseparable from bourgeois capitalism—a system entirely expressed, for Genet, by
its police. Drawing on Deleuze and Guattari, Guy Hocquenghem, in Homosexual Desire (Le désir homosexuel), analyzes the sexualization of the anus as a
revolutionary return to the stage of nondifferentiated desire that precedes the
establishment of personhood and social order. For Hocquenghem, this entails a radical destabilization of the subject: "It is no longer I who am speaking
when the desiring use of the anus asserts itself" (89) ["Ce n'est plus moi qui
parle quand l'usage désirant de l'anus s'impose" (68)]. Asserting such desire, as
Genet's narrator does by making it appear publicly at the very heart of the system (the police station) immediately threatens the social and symbolic order. As
Hocquenghem writes:

> Homosexual desire is related in particular to the pre-personal state of de-
> sire. . . . The direct manifestation of homosexual desire stands in contrast
> to the relations of identity, the necessary roles imposed by the Oedipus
> complex in order to ensure the reproduction of society. (92)

> [Le désir homosexuel se rapporte particulièrement à l'état pré-personnel
> du désir. . . . La manifestation immédiate du désir homosexuel s'oppose
> aux rapports d'identité, aux rôles nécessaires qu'impose Œdipe pour as-
> surer la reproduction de la société. (71–72)]

For Genet, a harmless little object such as a used tube of Vaseline can threaten
to undo the whole system by bringing back inside what had been abjected to an
inexpressible outside. This episode, situated at the beginning of the text, announces Genet's unraveling of binary oppositions. As we shall see in the next

section, he uses the relationship between police and thieves as the ideal site for subverting such oppositions.

Interestingly, the narrator's account of the incident is interrupted by an image, the memory of his encounter with a destitute old woman he identifies as a thief just out of jail, and who, he fantasizes, was the mother he never knew. To honor her, he imagines the opposite of the usual displays of filial devotion:

> It did not take long for my mind to replace these customary marks of tenderness by just any other gesture, even the vilest and most contemptible, which I empowered to mean as much as the kisses, or the tears, or the flowers.
>
> "I'd be glad to slobber over her," I thought, overflowing with love. . . . "To slobber over her hair or vomit into her hands. But I would adore that thief who is my mother." (21; translation modified)

> [Il fallut peu de temps à mon esprit pour qu'il remplaçât ces marques habituelles de la tendresse par n'importe quel geste et même par les plus décriés, par les plus vils, que je chargeais de signifier autant que les baisers, ou les larmes, ou les fleurs.
>
> — Je me contenterais de baver sur elle, pensais-je, en débordant d'amour. . . . De baver sur ses cheveux ou de vomir dans ses mains. Mais je l'adorerais cette voleuse qui est ma mère. (22)]

According to Kristeva, the abject corresponds to the need to separate from the maternal in order to enter the symbolic. The scene above reads like a reversal of the abjection of the maternal, as the narrator appears to reclaim his abjected mother, and threatens to undo the symbolic by returning to the point of its articulation. It is no surprise that the return of nondifferentiated desire immediately triggers, in the text, the return of the abjected mother. As Genet writes: "The tube of vaseline whose purpose is rather well known to you, summoned up the face of her who, during a reverie that moved through the dark alleys of the city, was the most cherished of mothers" (21; translation modified) ["Le tube de vaseline, dont la destination vous est assez connue, aura fait surgir le visage de celle qui durant une rêverie se poursuivant le long des ruelles noires de la ville, fut la mère la plus chérie" (22)]. For Genet, they both represent the same fundamental threat to the system.

But how does Genet articulate the relation between his abject world of disease, vermin, and homosexuality on the one hand, and the system that came into existence by the act of abjection on the other? As we begin to see in the episode of the tube of Vaseline, his rhetorical strategy in *Journal du voleur* consists in exposing the structural role of exclusion and the founding absence within the system, his own absence:

> Excluded by my birth and tastes from the social order, I was not aware of its diversity. I wondered at its perfect coherence, which rejected me. I was astounded by so rigorous an edifice whose details united against me. Nothing in the world was irrelevant: the stars on a general's sleeve, the stock-market quotations, the olive harvest, the style of the judiciary, the wheat exchange, flower beds . . . Nothing. This order, fearful and feared, whose details were all perfectly connected, had a meaning: my exile. (182; translation modified)

> [Exclu par ma naissance et mes goûts d'un ordre social, je n'en distinguais pas la diversité. J'en admirais la parfaite cohérence qui me refusait. J'étais stupéfait devant un édifice si rigoureux dont les détails se comprenaient contre moi. Rien au monde n'était insolite: les étoiles sur la manche d'un général, les cours de Bourse, la cueillette des olives, le style judiciaire, le marché du grain, les parterres de fleurs . . . Rien. Cet ordre redoutable, redouté, dont tous les détails étaient en connexion exacte avait un sens: mon exil. (192–93)]

In this passage, Genet does not simply remind us that in the Western, bourgeois society he describes, the military, the economy, and the law are exclusionary institutions; he wouldn't be saying anything his readers didn't already know. Rather, Genet's narrator becomes the locus of the system's coherence and meaning. Coherence and meaning are, of course, what makes a system a system, that without which there is no system. And that coherence, that meaning, are located outside the system's boundaries. In other words, the narrator represents the nonorigin, the founding absence, something like a Derridean trace. By constantly reminding the system of his shifting existence, mostly through his crimes and repeated deportations, the narrator prevents its closure and threatens its boundaries. He is, in a word, abject.

A paradox remains, however. The thief, the *Journal*'s narrator, claims to represent the personification of the abject, but can one represent or textually embody the abject? Indeed, the abject is precisely that which cannot be represented without threatening to lift the system's constitutive boundary and, therefore, risking the collapse of the symbolic order. As a representation, the abject can only figure the ritualized repetition of the act of abjection, that is, the reinforcement of the boundary.[23] The figures of leprosy and lice developed in the text should then be read as stages within a representational strategy that must be more globally disruptive if Genet is to solve what Bergen identifies as "the problematic of expressing the other, the doomed element, in the presence of a linguistic garb that kills what it talks about, and only gives form and meaning to the normalized part of reality" ["la problématique du dire l'autre du langage, la part maudite, en présence d'un vêtement langagier qui tue ce dont il parle et ne met en forme et en sens que la part normée du réel" (49)]. The term "garb"— *vêtement* in the original French—is particularly well chosen since it is really a question of "putting on" a language thus reduced to being a collection of empty signifiers.[24] The result of Genet's appropriation of the rhetoric of disease and infection is the contamination of language itself.

Crossing Metaphorical Borders, or Contaminating Language

We discussed how Genet reverses the figures of the louse and the tube of Vaseline to turn them into precious emblems. I mentioned that this technique of inversion is typical of Genet's poetics. The very opening of *Journal du voleur* is a perfect example of such inversion, which is at the same time stylistic and sexual because of the desire that triggers the production of Genet's language. Here, then, is how the novel opens:

> Convicts' garb is striped pink and white. If it was at my heart's bidding that I chose the universe wherein I delight, I at least have the power of finding therein the many meanings I wish to find: *there is a close relationship between flowers and convicts*. The fragility and delicacy of the former are of the same nature as the brutal insensitivity of the latter.* Should I have to portray a convict—or a criminal—I shall so bedeck him with flowers that, as he disappears beneath them, he will himself become a flower, a gigantic and new one. (9; original emphasis; translation modified)

> [Le vêtement des forçats est rayé rose et blanc. Si, commandé par mon coeur l'univers où je me complais, je l'élus, ai-je le pouvoir au moins d'y découvrir les nombreux sens que je veux: *il existe donc un rapport étroit entre les fleurs et les bagnards*. La fragilité, la délicatesse des premières sont de même nature que la brutale insensibilité des autres.* Que j'aie à représenter un forçat—ou un criminel—je le parerai de tant de fleurs que lui-

même disparaissant sous elles en deviendra une autre, géante, nouvelle. (9; original emphasis)]

The asterisk sends the reader to the following footnote: "*My excitement is the oscillation from one to the other" (9) ["*Mon émoi c'est l'oscillation des unes aux autres" (9)]. And Genet adds a little later: "The material evokes, both by its colors and roughness, certain flowers whose petals are slightly fuzzy, which detail is sufficient for me to associate most naturally the idea of strength and shame with what is precious and fragile" (10; translation modified) ["Outre ses teintes, par sa rugosité, l'étoffe évoque certaines fleurs dont les pétales sont légèrement velus, détail suffisant pour qu'à l'idée de force et de honte j'associe le plus naturellement précieux et fragile" (10)]. More than the expression of sexual desire and Genet's propensity to shock his readers, his poetic strategy hints at the co-constitutive nature of opposites, and even their mythical, or presymbolic, nondifferentiation. By bringing into contact fragility and strength, delicacy and insensitivity, and so on, Genet makes both terms of these dichotomies infect each other.

The link between "convicts" and "flowers" exists only insofar as Genet makes it up. His narrator reclaims the status of subject with the "power" to produce meaning, or make sense. In other words, he compromises with the symbolic structure, but ultimately to hijack it. While a normalizing language would demand the separation of the words "convicts" and "flowers," that doesn't mean, however, that they cannot be brought together as metaphors for one another. Theoretically at least, all such associations are possible, and they don't necessarily entail a radical destabilization of language. But some associations, like that of "convicts" and "flowers," normally fall outside of meaning; they are meaningless or absurd or mad. Genet, on the other hand, endows his word association with meaning. In the text, the metaphorical coupling of "convicts" and "flowers" results in the mutual infection of each term, and signifies the transformation of the system that demanded that, put together, they produce no meaning. The structure in which Genet's metaphor has a meaning cannot be the same as the one that forbids it. For Sartre, Genet "wants to name, not in order to *designate* but to *transform*" (280; original emphasis) ["il veut nommer, non pour *désigner* mais pour *transformer*" (314; original emphasis)], in a fundamentally viral operation the former calls a "verbal disease" (281) ["la maladie verbale" (315)]. The opening passage of *Journal du voleur* suggests that the viral infection occurs first of all from signifier to signifier.

Moreover, the mutual contamination of opposites necessarily implies that there is a threat at the very border that articulates them as such. More directly perhaps than in his earlier work, Genet problematizes the idea of the border in

Journal du voleur. A large part of this text tells the story of its narrator's travels throughout Europe, and images of borders are many. The narrator crosses them, back and forth, sometimes illegally while smuggling opium or counterfeit money, often as he is deported from one country to the next. What ultimately emerges from these repeated instances of border crossing in the text is the idea of the border as *pliure,* or line of articulation of a series of interchangeable dichotomies: the inside/outside separation, the subject/object domination, the mutual repulsion of clean and unclean, of healthy and sick. Genet's poetic enterprise underscores the mutual dependency of the two terms of these dichotomies and allows him to act at the (fictitious) line that articulates them—the border.

Throughout the text, Genet insists on how easy it is for police and thieves to switch their positions back and forth, and avers that the possibility of that inversion is originary, yet repressed—as hinted by the tube of Vaseline. Such oscillation is made possible by what he calls "[a] verbal kinship" ["une parenté verbale"] and "a kind of secret connection unknown to the world, the kind which permits a shepherdess to chat familiarly with a king of France" (175) ["une sorte de relation secrète, ignorée du monde, celle qui permet à une bergère de tutoyer un roi de France" (185)]. For instance, when the narrator puts on the cape he stole from a customs officer with whom he just had sex for money, he feels "a kind of presentiment of a conclusion wherein law and outlaw merge, one lurking beneath the other but each feeling, with a touch of nostalgia, the virtue of its opposite" (51; translation modified) ["comme le pressentiment d'une conclusion où la loi et le hors-la-loi se confondent, l'un se dissimulant sous l'autre mais éprouvant avec un peu de nostalgie la vertu de son contraire" (54)]. It is precisely when repulsion turns into nostalgia that the social and symbolic order is in the greatest of dangers—and when the narrator's excitement is the highest. This is the time when the presymbolic moment of nondifferentiation, the a-memorial past before the founding act of abjection, resurfaces in his consciousness.

At one point, the narrator has an affair with a man named Bernardini who is both a cop and a thief. This relationship gives the narrator the opportunity to deepen his awareness of the fragility of each man's position. Using a vocabulary that emphasizes the role homosexuality plays in that process of disruption, Genet writes: "I felt as if I were penetrating to the very heart of the police. I must have wandered deep into it for a detective to be ironical with me about his function. However, it seems to me that this joke revealed to us the absurdity of our reciprocal situation" (195; translation modified) ["J'avais le sentiment de pénétrer au plus intime de la police. Il fallait qu'en effet je fusse égaré profondément en elle pour qu'un policier ironise avec moi de sa fonction. Toute-fois, me semble-t-il, ce jeu nous indiquait dérisoire notre réciproque condition" (207)]. Note the singular "situation," indicating that it is really one and the same. And on murder Genet adds:

> I respected the police. They can kill. Not at a distance and by proxy, but with their hands. Their murders, though ordered, derive nonetheless from a particular, individual will implying, along with its decision, the re-sponsibility of the murderer. The policeman is taught to kill. . . . The po-lice come from a similar school, just as the young heroes from Dickens come from a school for pickpockets. (196–97)

> [Je respectais la police. Elle peut tuer. Non à distance et par procuration mais de sa main. Ses meurtres, s'ils sont ordonnés, n'en relèvent pas moins d'une volonté particulière, individuelle, impliquant, avec sa décision, la responsabilité du meurtrier. Au policier on enseigne à tuer. . . . La police semble d'une semblable école comme les jeunes héros de Dickens des écoles de vol à la tire. (208–9)]

In addition, the description of the police station directly echoes the un-wholesome world of the narrator's gang of thieves, prostitutes, and beggars. In the world of the police, one can also feel "an atmosphere of sullen rancor, of foul infamy, and it gives me [the narrator] pleasure to know that these big strapping fellows are breathing in it and that it is corrupting them, that it is evilly corrod-ing their minds" (197) ["une atmosphère de sourde rancoeur, de crapuleuse in-fâmie, que j'aime savoir respirée par ces costauds qu'elle corrompt, dont elle corrode méchamment l'esprit" (209)]. The metaphors of sickness and corrup-tion, both metaphors of exclusion, are now redirected against the most symbolic representatives (for Genet, at least) of the system that had produced them in the first place. Genet the louse can now call the ideal cop "the perfect insect" (197) ["l'insecte parfait" (209)]. The (metaphorical) border as *pliure* thus underscores the specular relation between order and disorder.

According to the same logic, the police state at its most advanced level, Nazi Germany, corresponds to the outlaw state: "a camp organized by bandits" (123) ["un camp organisé par des bandits" (131)]. When traveling there, the thief finds himself on the side of order:

> I was excited at being free amidst an entire people that had been placed on the index. . . . "It's a race of thieves," I thought to myself. "If I steal here, I perform no singular deed that might fulfill me. I obey the customary or-

der; I do not destroy it. I am not committing evil. I am not upsetting anything. The outrageous is impossible. I am stealing in the void." (123)

[J'étais ému d'être libre au milieu d'un peuple mis à l'index. . . . C'est un
peuple de voleurs, sentais-je en moi même. Si je vole ici je n'accomplis aucune action singulière et qui puisse me réaliser mieux: j'obéis à l'ordre
habituel. Je ne le détruis pas. Je ne commets pas le mal, je ne dérange rien.
Le scandale est impossible. Je vole à vide. (131)]

As soon as the thief crosses the border into Nazi Germany, all values and positions are automatically reversed. But because of its ambiguous status as a criminal state, Germany points toward an apocalyptic resolution, when dichotomies
cease to exist. The narrator observes: "Only Germany, in Hitler's time, succeeded
in being both Police and Crime. This masterly synthesis of opposites, this block
of truth, was frightful, and charged with a magnetism that will continue to per-
turb us for a long time" (189; translation modified) ["Les Allemands seuls, à
l'époque de Hitler, réussirent à être à la fois la Police et le Crime. Cette magis-
trale synthèse des contraires, ce bloc de vérité étaient épouvantables, chargés
d'un magnétisme qui nous affolera longtemps" (200)]. Nazis, in fact, are mostly
of interest to Genet as invaders and destroyers of French institutions; but as another novel, *Pompes funèbres,* indicates, he really prefers French militiamen who
embody betrayal and duplicity better than Nazis could.[25]

In *Journal du voleur,* an episode involving the narrator and a border guard
literally situates the articulation of opposites at the very locus of its origin—
the boundary. In this episode, involving homosexuality, crime, and duplicity,
the narrator seduces a Spanish border guard—on duty—and has sex with him
while smugglers enter the country with impunity. By doing so, the narrator
appropriates the power of the border guard and gains control over the boundary
articulating inside and outside. As he remarks: "I realized that it was up to me
whether or not the smugglers landed safely" (171) ["je compris qu'il ne tenait
qu'à moi que les fraudeurs abordassent sans danger" (180)]. Genet's sexuality,
that is, one of the reasons for his social exclusion, is the very tool with which he
affects and corrupts the authority in charge of the border. And when the border
guard hears the smugglers and decides not to intervene, his authority has effectively been dissolved. In this episode, sexual inversion, which brought convicts
and flowers together at the outset of the novel, is the key element in the disruption of the "normal" law/outlaw relation and, consequently, of the normalizing
system entirely contained in this dichotomy. Genet can logically conclude:

Betrayal, theft and homosexuality are the basic subjects of this book.
There is a relationship among them which, though not always apparent,

at least, it seems to me, recognizes a kind of vascular exchange between my taste for betrayal and theft and my loves. (171)

[La trahison, le vol et l'homosexualité sont les sujets essentiels de ce livre. Un rapport existe entre eux, sinon apparent toujours, du moins me semble-t-il reconnaître une sorte d'échange vasculaire entre mon goût pour la trahison, le vol et mes amours. (181)]

It is precisely by reclaiming the very qualities used to identify him as an outlaw that the narrator incorporates the qualities of the border guard, while the latter becomes complicit in an illegal act: "I granted him the loveliest of my nights. Not so that he might be happy but that I might take upon myself—and deliver him from—his own ignominy" (171) ["Je lui accordai la plus belle de mes nuits. Non pour qu'il soit heureux mais afin de me charger—et de l'en délivrer—de sa propre ignominie" (181)].

For the thief, to wear a policeman's outfit also represents a symbolic disruption of the law/outlaw dichotomy. After the narrator steals the custom officer's cape, in the episode I mentioned earlier, he notes: "I wrapped myself up in it in order to return to the hotel, and I knew the happiness of the equivocal, not yet the joy of betrayal, though the insidious confusion which would make me deny fundamental oppositions was already forming" (32) ["Je m'en enveloppai pour revenir à l'hôtel, et je connus le bonheur de l'équivoque, non encore la joie de la trahison, mais déjà la confusion s'établissait, insidieuse, qui me ferait nier les oppositions fondamentales" (34)]. Yet the simple, specular reversal of the inside/outside dichotomy isn't sufficient in itself to "deny fundamental oppositions," for such oppositions only reconstitute themselves in the end. When, near the conclusion of the text, Genet writes: "I will cease to be the judge and the accused" (245) ["Je cesserai d'être le juge et l'accusé" (261)], he implies the possibility of reaching a point when he could neutralize the binary dynamic of specular relations, when he wouldn't be on either side of the border but rather exactly *at* the border, neither subject nor object.

Literal Borders

The crossing of literal borders as well is often described with great lyricism in *Journal du voleur,* as in the following passage:

Almost always alone, though aided by an ideal companion, I crossed other borders. My emotion was always equally great. I crossed Alps of all kinds. . . . Fought by the wind, by the cold, by the thorns, by November, I reached a summit behind which was Italy. In order to reach it I faced monsters hidden by the night or revealed by it. (113; translation modified)

[Presque toujours seul, mais aidé d'un idéal compagnon, je traversai d'autre frontières. Mon émotion était toujours aussi grande. Je franchis toutes sortes d'Alpes . . . . Combattu par le vent, par le froid, par les ronces, par novembre, j'atteignis un sommet derrière quoi était l'Italie. Pour la gagner j'affrontais des monstres cachés par la nuit ou révélés par elle. (120)]

This emotion is such because something primordial is at stake in the crossing of a border, as if each such crossing gave a material existence to the oscillation between "convicts" and "flowers" in the opening.

Before addressing the nature of borders, it may be necessary to remember why the narrator crosses them so often. For this textual outlaw, crossing a border is seldom a positive act motivated by, say, curiosity for the country he is entering, but rather a negative one, defined by his departure from the other country, as in: "The landscape of France put Belgium behind me" (255) ["Le paysage de France reculait derrière moi la Belgique" (271)]. He goes from place to place according to the will of the police, expelled from one country, refused entry by another, and so on:

My ragged clothing, filthy face and long, dirty hair frightened the customs officers, who would not let me disembark. Back in Spain, I decided to go by way of Ceuta; when I got there, I was put into jail for four days and had to go back to where I had come from. (83)

[Mes vêtements en loques, ma figure crasseuse, mes cheveux longs et sales effrayèrent les douaniers qui m'empêchèrent de débarquer. De retour en Espagne je décidai de passer par Ceuta: en y arrivant on m'emprisonna quatre jours et je dus retourner d'où j'étais parti. (88)]

And later:

The port authority in Corfu refused to let me stay. Before I could leave again, they made me spend the night on the boat I had hired to bring me. Afterward it was Serbia. Afterward Austria. Czechoslovakia. Poland, where I tried to circulate counterfeit zlotys. Everywhere it was the same: robbery, prison, and, from every one of these countries, expulsion. (92)

[A Corfou les autorités du port me refusent de séjourner. Sur la barque que j'ai louée pour m'amener, ils m'obligent à passer la nuit avant de repartir. Après c'est la Serbie. Après l'Autriche. La Tchécoslovaquie. La Pologne où je cherche à écouler de faux zlotys. C'est partout le vol, la prison, et de chacun de ces pays l'expulsion. (98)]

There are too many examples to quote them all.

In *Journal du voleur,* the opening depictions of convicts sent to penal colonies overseas bring a physical reality to the border, while exemplifying the idea that criminal elements must be expelled from the body politic toward an unwholesome and mysterious outside.[26] The *bagne,* the hard-labor camps in Guiana, long enjoyed an undisputed supremacy in the French imagery of crime as the evil flip side of civil society. When sent there, a convict crossed something like a primordial border, figured here by the ocean. Because it is extraterritorial in nature, the ocean is often linked to lawlessness in Genet's poetic universe.[27] By extension, the harbor finds itself at the point of articulation between inside and outside, law and outlaw, *monde* and *immonde.* The harbor is a place of transit for infections and for individuals rhetorically constructed as infectious, such as criminals, smugglers, prostitutes, deviants, and especially spies and traitors. In *Querelle de Brest* that harbor was Brest, in *Journal du voleur* it is Tangiers: "I thought about Tangiers, whose proximity fascinated me, as did the glamor of the city, that haunt, rather, of traitors" (71) ["Je songeais à Tanger dont la proximité me fascinait et le prestige de cette ville, plutôt repère de traîtres" (76)].

Genet is fully aware, however, that Tangiers is a construct, a paranoid fantasy within the European cultural imagination, and that is precisely why he chooses to embrace it, just as he did the equally fantasmatic images of leprosy and lice. Because the police—defined as a "concentrated delegation of the world" (20) ["délégation concentrée du monde" (21)]—are contained in language—"the style of the judiciary" (182) ["le style judiciaire" (193)]—the narrator seeks to identify less with betrayal proper than with its most universally recognized sign, Tangiers:

> I would have liked to embark for Tangiers. *Movies* and *novels* have made of this city a fearful place, a kind of dive where gamblers haggle over the secret plans of all the armies in the world. From the Spanish coast, Tangiers *seemed* to me a *fabulous* city. It was the very *symbol* of treason. . . . [T]his city *represented* Treason so accurately, so magnificently, that I felt I was bound to land there. (83; my emphasis)

> [J'aurais voulu m'embarquer pour Tanger. Les *films* et les *romans* ont fait de cette ville un lieu terrible, une sorte de tripot où les joueurs marchan-

dent les plans secrets de toutes les armées du monde. De la côte espag-
nole, Tanger me *paraissait* une cité *fabuleuse*. Elle était le *symbole* même de
la trahison. . . . [C]ette ville pour moi *représentait* si bien, si magnifique-
ment la Trahison que c'est là, me semblait-il, que je ne pourrais qu'aborder. (88–89; my emphasis)]

The vocabulary of fiction used by Genet indicates that what attracts him to Tangiers is its function as sign or symbol, its qualities as a magnificent representation. And if Treason, with a capital *T,* is a construct, then so is its positive opposite, Loyalty. The campy tone of the passage further emphasizes the idea of
artificiality and denaturalizes the construction of treason as evil and loyalty as
good.

In the text, the themes of espionage and treason allow Genet to deal more
directly with the idea of contaminating the body politic. The spy/virus infil-
trates/infects a country/body in order to weaken it. Not surprisingly, the spy
who most fascinates Genet is the absolute spy, the one who betrays for the sake
of betraying, without any concern for loyalty to one side or the other. The reason for Genet's attraction does not lie in the gratuitousness of the act, however—
for a crime, he avers, must be motivated by interest; instead, it lies in the fact
that such a spy would be the embodiment of duplicity, the absolute foreign body,
the heterogeneous by definition, the perpetual outsider within. Spying, in short,
testifies to the instability of borders; hence the fascination with Tangiers.

Because it is both a harbor and a border town, Tangiers is a place where dichotomies, or "fundamental oppositions," are articulated. In fact, Tangiers is not
really *at* the border; it *is* the border, in the sense that it is constructed by Genet
(and by the European cultural imagination within which Genet writes) as extraterritorial. Situated at the entry (or exit) of the Mediterranean, that is, the
cradle of Western civilization, it represents the boundary of that civilization. Essentially a cosmopolitan city, it is neither really African, nor really European. It
conjures up the same sorts of images as Constantinople, its Eastern counterpart
(neither really Asian, nor really European). The West projects and channels its
fear of invasion and contamination on such shady and seemingly stateless cities.
Like all borders, Tangiers is intangible. It is constructed as a place which is not
really one, as a kind of no-man's-land, albeit one populated by creatures whose
humanity seems very much in doubt. As the textual embodiment of the border,
it can only be a dangerous place.

As Genet insists on the fictional nature of Tangiers, he reminds us that this is
the case of all borders. Indeed, what is a border, if not a theoretical line without
any material existence? It is actually impossible to freeze the moment when one

is exactly at the border, and not on either side of it. Jacques Derrida, in *Glas*, writes about a "frontier all the more mysterious, concealed in the crossing, because it is abstract, legal, ideal . . . that is, the invisible, artificial, nonexistent line, that you transgress without seeing, with a single step, in a limit instant, like noon, no, that you do not pass presently but that you are going to pass, that you have passed" (189) ["une frontière d'autant plus mystérieuse, dérobée au franchissement, qu'elle est abstaite, légale, idéale . . . c'est-à-dire invisible, artificielle, inexistante, qu'on transgresse sans la voir, d'un seul pas, en un instant limite, comme midi, non qu'on ne passe pas présentement mais qu'on va passer, qu'on a passée" (212)].

The only way to freeze such a noninstant, when one crosses a nonentity, is to construct both of them textually in the novel. Although the border may have no tangible existence, it defines nonetheless what it outlines; it gives its meaning to what is essentially a fictional representation—and, at the same time, threatens it. Simply put: there is no country without borders. But, as Butler notes: "excluded sites come to bound the 'human' as its constitutive outside, and to haunt those boundaries as the persistent possibility of their disruption and rearticulation" (*Bodies That Matter*, 8). The very condition of the system's existence is, simultaneously and inevitably, the reminder of its possible end. Hence Genet's emotion when entering, not a real country, but a representation of one that would not exist without him: "The crossing of borders and the excitement it arouses in me were to enable me to apprehend directly the essence of the nation I was entering. I would penetrate less into a country than inside an image" (49; translation modified) ["Le passage des frontières et cette émotion qu'il me cause devaient me permettre d'appréhender directement l'essence de la nation où j'entrais. Je pénétrais moins dans un pays qu'à l'intérieur d'une image" (51)]. Hence, also, the dual position of the border, both central and peripheral. With no intrinsic value, it is what makes it possible to say that there is value, that there is a positive and a negative, an inside and an outside, a subject and an object[28]—precisely because it cannot be reduced to either term of these founding dichotomies. For Derrida, the crossing of this limit is "the punctual instant, unseizable but revolutionary . . . when . . . the opposition is lifted, the limit suspended, the inside and the outside pass into one another" (*Glas*, 190) ["l'instant ponctuel, insaisissable mais révolutionnaire . . . où . . . l'opposition est levée, la limite suspendue, le dedans et le dehors passent l'un dans l'autre" (213)]. Ultimately, Genet will try to represent the crossing of the border and construct himself as the natural, presymbolic, abject inhabitant of the no-man's-land. This sends us back to the question I raised earlier: How can the abject be represented when the very possibility of representation demands that it be expelled?

In the text, when the narrator crosses the border from Czechoslovakia to Poland, Genet's poetics may give readers an idea about how to solve (rather than answer) that question. The crossing involves an original rejection, the impossible moment itself, and the thief's emotion when he knows he finds himself at the mythical time and place of creation of an order:

The tapestry known as "Lady with the Unicorn" excited me for reasons I shall not attempt to go into here. But when I crossed the border from Czechoslovakia into Poland, it was noon, in the summer. The ideal line ran through a field of ripe rye. . . . I was with another fellow who, like me, had been expelled by the Czech police, but I very soon lost sight of him; perhaps he had strayed off behind a bush or wanted to get rid of me. He disappeared. The rye field was bounded on the Polish side by a wood at whose edge was nothing but motionless birches; on the Czech side, by another wood, but of fir trees. I remained a long time squatting at the edge, intently wondering what lay hidden in the field. If I crossed it were customs officers hidden in the rye? Invisible hares must have been running through it. I was uneasy. At noon, beneath a pure sky, all nature was offering me a puzzle, and offering it to me blandly.

"If something happens," I said to myself, "it will be the appearance of a unicorn. Such a moment and such a place can only produce a unicorn."

Fear and the kind of emotion I always feel when I cross a border, conjured up at noon, beneath a leaden sun, the first fairyland. I ventured forth into that golden sea as one enters the water. I went through the rye standing up. I advanced slowly, surely, with the certainty of being the heraldic character for whom a natural blazon has been formed: azure, field of gold, sun, forests. . . .

When I got to the birches, I was in Poland. An enchantment of another order was about to be offered me. The "Lady with the Unicorn" is to me the lofty expression of this crossing the line at noontide. (47–48; translation modified)

[La tapisserie intitulée "La Dame à la Licorne" m'a bouleversé pour des raisons que je n'entreprendrai pas ici d'énumérer. Mais quand je passai de Tchécoslovaquie en Pologne, la frontière, c'était un midi, l'été. La ligne idéale traversait un champ de seigle mûr. . . . J'étais avec un autre garçon expulsé comme moi par la police tchèque, mais je le perdis de vue très vite, peut-être s'égara-t-il derrière un bosquet ou voulut-il m'abandonner: il disparut. Ce champ de seigle était bordé du côté polonais par un bois dont l'orée n'était que de bouleaux immobiles. Du côté tchèque d'un autre bois, mais de sapins. Longtemps je restai accroupi au bord, attentif à me demander ce que recélait ce champ, si je le traversai quels douaniers les seigles dissimulaient. Des lièvres invisibles devaient le parcourir. J'étais inquiet. A midi, sous un ciel pur, la nature entière me proposait une énigme, et me la proposait avec suavité.

— S'il se passe quelque chose, me disais-je, c'est l'apparition d'une licorne.

La peur, et la sorte d'émotion que j'éprouve toujours quand je passe une frontière, suscitaient à midi, sous un soleil de plomb la première féérie. Je me hasardai dans cette mer dorée comme on entre dans l'eau. Debout je traversai les seigles. Je m'avançai lentement, sûrement, avec la certitude d'être le personnage héraldique pour qui s'est formé un blason naturel: azur, champ d'or, soleil, forêts. . . .

En arrivant aux bouleaux, j'étais en Pologne. Un enchantement d'un autre ordre m'allait être proposé. La "Dame à la Licorne" m'est l'expression hautaine de ce passage de la ligne à midi. (50–51)]

Genet insists on the fact that the crossing takes place at noon. Noon, just like midnight, divides time in two, except that noon is in the middle of the day, in broad daylight. At the beginning of the novel, Genet had already written: "The penal colony is in the sun. Everything takes place in a cruel light which I cannot refrain from choosing as the sign of lucidity" (11, note; translation modified) ["Le bagne est au soleil. C'est dans une lumière cruelle que tout se passe, et je ne puis m'empêcher de la choisir comme signe de la lucidité" (12, note)]. What midnight conceals, noon reveals. In this case, the narrator reveals the cut between inside and outside, that is, the very time and place when an order is created, the "enchantment of another order." But he also reveals that the border guard, whom one could only imagine as terrible, is in fact a sweet and harmless unicorn, really a myth. Crossing the border, then, seems much less dangerous than expected.

Furthermore, the unicorn can be read as a symbol of original plenitude. It conveys a multilayered intertext, including the legendary origin of the Plantagenêt family: the unicorn, the broom (in French, *genêt*), the creation of a name, the inauguration of a line, of a national and heraldic order. In *Glas*, Derrida reminds us that it was once believed that the horns of the unicorn were a universal counterpoison (192 [216]). In Genet's text, the unicorn, a creature of the border, represents a return to the presymbolic, that is, something like the counterpoison for metaphors, and the moment when the separation of inside and outside, of healthy and sick get neutralized: it is the sweet counterpart of the abject. In addition to this specific passage, Genet uses numerous medieval references to figure the return to the a-memorial. There are the narrator's identification with Gilles de Rais, for example, and the connotations of leprosy we discussed earlier. This use of ancient intertexts is explicitly acknowledged by Genet, who writes: "*I make my way through genealogical strata, the Renaissance, the Middle Ages, Carolingian, Merovingian, Byzantine and Roman times, the epics and invasions, in order to arrive at the Fable where all creation is possible*" (168; original emphasis) ["*je traverse les couches généalogiques, la Renaissance, le moyen âge, les époques carolingienne, mérovingienne, byzantine, romaine, les épopées, les invasions, afin de parvenir à la Fable où toute création est possible*" (178; original emphasis)]. This movement points toward a mythical past, a fabulous origin, when the original act of exclusion took place and language was inaugurated.[29] By embodying the excluded element, the narrator's abjection is the foundation of the system. He is the origin of meaning, what gives the system its coherence, but also, as we have seen, the reminder of that system's inherent fragility, the lurking threat of meaninglessness.

Is the narrator, therefore, sentenced to perpetual movement? By the very fact that the text figures the neutralization of the subject/object dichotomy and attempts to represent the abject, it reasserts subject and object and the act of abjection (without which there would be no representation). In other words, Genet seems to use the "natural" function of language. Does he even have a choice? Yet, faced with the impossibility of escaping the symbolic order, rather than naturalizing it, he keeps exposing its hidden origin and so reveals the instability of its borders.

Finally, everything for Genet is a movement toward a saintliness he shall never reach; unless, of course, saintliness is in fact in the movement itself:

> I call saintliness not a state, but the moral process that leads me to it. It is the ideal point of a morality which I cannot talk about since I do not see it. It withdraws when I approach it. I desire it and fear it. This process may appear stupid. Yet, though painful, it is joyful. It's a queen. It foolishly assumes the figure of a Carolina carried off in her skirts and screaming with happiness. (215; translation modified)

> [Je nomme sainteté, non un état, mais la démarche morale qui m'y conduit. C'est le point idéal d'une morale dont je ne puis parler car je ne l'aperçois pas. Il s'éloigne quand je m'approche de lui. Je le désire et le redoute. Cette démarche peut paraître imbécile. Cependant encore que

douloureuse, elle est joyeuse. C'est une folle. Sottement elle prend la figure d'une Caroline enlevée sur ses jupes et hurlant de bonheur. (228)]

If, as the passage indicates, (the movement toward) saintliness is best represented by the image of a Carolina, a screaming drag queen, then such saintliness is defined by the destabilization of binary oppositions (in this case the binary system of gender, but, as I posited at the outset, all such dichotomies contain the system that produced them). Saintliness, then, is the movement toward the undoing of order, and that is precisely what characterizes Genet's poetics. His ultimate and unreachable goal is to embody the poetic process itself, and he asks: "When might I finally leap into the heart of the image, be myself the light which carries it to your eyes? When might I be in the heart of poetry?" (215) ["Quand pourrais-je enfin bondir au coeur de l'image, être moi-même la lumière qui la porte jusqu'à vos yeux? Quand serais-je au coeur de la poésie?" (229)]. The somewhat unsettling use of the conditional mood in these sentences suggests that there might be no other answers to these questions than the questions themselves.

In his book *Homos,* Leo Bersani describes Genet's project as "the ambitious intention of imagining a form of revolt that has no relation whatsoever to the laws, categories, and values it would contest and, ideally, destroy" (152). And he adds that "Genet's use of his culture's dominant terms . . . are [sic] designed not to rework or to subvert those terms, but to exploit their potential for erasing cultural relationality itself (that is, the very preconditions for subversive repositionings and defiant repetitions)" (153). Unlike Bataille, Bersani sees Genet's perceived refusal to communicate as positive.[30] My reading of *Journal du voleur* leads me to a different conclusion than Bersani's (or Bataille's for that matter). I agree that Genet points toward a neutralization of dichotomies and of the system that rests on them. I do not agree, however, that such a move amounts to "erasing cultural relationality itself"—quite the contrary.

To begin with, what Bersani calls "cultural relationality" is the relation between opposites. But such a relation is, in fact, not relational at all since it is entirely self-contained—or, more accurately, it is entirely contained within the self; hence Genet's references to Guiana, the penal colony, as a part of himself, as when he writes: "Its abolition is so great a loss to me that I secretly recompose within me and for myself alone, a colony more vicious than that of Guiana" (11, note) ["Son abolition me prive à ce point qu'en moi-même et pour moi seul, secrètement, je recompose un bagne, plus méchant que celui de la Guyane" (11, note)]. It is precisely that inseparable nature of self and nonself that Genet seeks to expose.

Finally, as I have tried to show in my reading of border crossings, Genet ends up positioning himself at a theoretical in-between. But the in-between can only be represented by default, that is, by a constant movement of oscillation between the two poles. Genet's disruption of binary oppositions, then, does not and cannot take the absolute, nihilistic form of fascism, a theoretical possibility that was suggested earlier. What made Nazi Germany monstrous was that it embodied its dual nature; it lived it as its permanent state. Originating in a fictional construction of the perfect order as a fusion of opposites, fascism attempted to realize its founding metaphor and, therefore, to end all metaphoricity. Logically, it produced a type of horror that exceeds representation. Genet, on the other hand, chooses to remain within the system of representation and condemns himself to a perpetual motion between opposites, rather than to a monstrous, Janus-like state. When he writes: "This book, *The Thief's Journal,* pursuit of the Impossible Nothingness" (94) ["Ce livre, 'Journal du Voleur': poursuite de l'Impossible Nullité" (100)], the emphasis should be on "Impossible." This doomed pursuit of nothingness doesn't mean, however, that one should talk about Genet's failure, as Bataille does—a reading Bersani opposes. In fact the very notions of failure and success become irrelevant for Genet, who is not interested in proposing a new hierarchized value system, but in destabilizing the idea of system. When Genet reclaims the logic of contamination that is metaphor, he extends that relational logic to all language, and he effectively prevents the reification of the social and symbolic order he inhabits. While it is really fascism that could be described (using Bersani's words for Genet's project) as "a form of revolt that has no relation whatsoever to the laws, categories, and values it would contest and, ideally, destroy" (152), Genet's politics, as elaborated in his many writings, statements, and actions from the 1960s until his death in 1986, particularly his support for the Black Panthers and the Palestinians, were essentially practices of cultural relationality and border crossing, literal and otherwise, in which solidarity comes not from sameness but from difference.[31]

To close this chapter, I shall return one last time to the opening of the novel. When Genet associates "convicts" and "flowers" and reveals, in each, the trace of its opposite, he thus resignifies traditional signifiers of gender. Genet feminizes the convicts and virilizes flowers, and he does it with a metaphor, that is, an act of linguistic contamination. By doing so he discloses that "convicts" are masculine and "flowers" are feminine only in the symbolic order that constructs them as such; that the survival of such an order demands that their metaphorical association produce no meaning; and finally that each term of a dichotomy is constituted by the exclusion of the other term, so that mutual contamination is always already at work. In order to destabilize the system entirely contained in all dichotomies, Genet consciously and actively assumes the normative discourse that constructs his sexuality in terms of inversion and infection. By doing so, he uses the novel to redefine the subject, not as that which must protect itself from contamination (it is always already contaminated), but, on the contrary, as the agent of contamination itself—as that which won't be territorialized.

4
∝

A Cultural History of AIDS Discourse

France and the United States

What AIDS Criticism?

AIDS is much more than a health crisis. Since 1981, when the first reports of the syndrome were published in medical journals, AIDS has triggered an extraordinary amount of representations of all kinds. To be sure, it isn't the first time that an infectious disease, perceived as inevitably fatal, has found itself saturated with what it is not supposed to have: meaning. Like many previous epidemics, the AIDS pandemic, too, has been largely constructed in and by several intersecting discourses: biomedical, sexual, racial, social, political, literary, et cetera. Unlike previous epidemics, however, the AIDS epidemic has developed at a time when information and communication technologies allow such discourses to spread with amazing efficiency and speed. It is no surprise, then, that textual criticism became an integral part of the fight against AIDS. Although the representations of AIDS and people living with HIV or AIDS are culturally and historically determined, and have changed over the years, many of the basic observations made by early American and British AIDS critics, the first to deal with the epidemic by critiquing its representations, remain operative today. In short, while AIDS representations must be historicized, the dominant ideology framing these representations from the outset of the epidemic hasn't changed; it has only been redeployed. Moreover, I find it analytically appropriate to read Hervé Guibert (in chapter 5) with and through the critical concepts that were elaborated around the time his novels were written and published, insofar as such criticism precisely addresses the types of AIDS representations that were predominant then, and which Guibert worked to undermine.

I shall then posit as my starting point the basic principles laid out by Douglas Crimp: "AIDS does not exist apart from the practices that conceptualize it, represent it, and respond to it. We know AIDS only in and through those practices"; Paula Treichler: "We cannot . . . look 'through' language to determine what AIDS 'really' is. Rather, we must explore the site where such determinations really occur and intervene at the point where meaning is created: in language"; and Simon Watney, for whom: "there is not in fact a single, unified 'truth' about AIDS, available to be represented directly and universally or, for that matter, to be misrepresented. . . . AIDS is not only a medical crisis on an unparalleled scale, it involves a crisis of representation itself."[1]

In addition, there exists a unique concern with terminology in the French context. The acronym *SIDA* (for "AIDS") has almost entirely disappeared from nonmedical or nonofficial writings, and the noun *sida* is now widely used. In her essay on Hervé Guibert, "Fantom Images," Emily Apter sees that specificity as significant in the literature of AIDS in France, but without analyzing it further. She writes: "The AIDS novel in France is the novel of *le sida*, spelled without capital letters. Do these differences in notation ·from the acronym and capitals of AIDS indicate a different construction of the illness? In all probability it does" (83). French journalist and author Hugo Marsan chooses to use the lower-case spelling "with the purely symbolic purpose to tone down the fantasmatic, tabloid-like connotations that have been too widely associated with the disease" ["dans le but, purement symbolique, d'atténuer le caractère fantasmatique et 'presse à scandales' qui s'est par trop attaché à la maladie"].[2] On the one hand, this may sound paradoxical since the acronym is closer to the original, supposedly neutral, medical terminology, and should therefore leave less room for cultural interference or noise. On the other hand, Marsan's reasoning mirrors the attitude of *dédramatisation* that prevailed in France in the early 1980s.[3] In *Une fin de siècle épidémique,* Isabelle Rieusset-Lemarié proposes to distinguish the two as follows:

> As it has shifted from the medical register to that of the media, the acronym *SIDA* . . . has tended to disappear and be replaced by the more commonplace "*sida*," written as a regular noun. . . . For precision's sake we have kept the form "*SIDA*" to denote acquired immune deficiency syn-

drome, as opposed to "*sida*," which we use only in its analogical, journalistic acception.

[En passant du registre médical au registre médiatique, le sigle SIDA . . . a eu tendance à disparaître au profit de sa banalisation en 'sida,' écrit comme un nom commun. . . . Pour plus de rigueur nous avons maintenu l'écriture "SIDA," lorsqu'il s'agit de désigner le syndrome d'immunodéficience acquise, par opposition à "sida" dont nous avons réservé l'emploi à son usage analogique médiatique. (140 n. 2)]

Rieusset-Lemarié's convention could actually be generalized. *SIDA*, then, would be used only in a purely denotative, medical function—provided that there could even be such a thing—while *sida* would be used for everything else, that is, the multiple crises triggered by the onset of AIDS and the many discourses attached to it. This distinction, however, is problematic to begin with if we admit that medical discourse is always already undermined by its founding metaphoricity.[4] It is therefore impossible to name a "real" disease in a supposedly untainted, discourse-free fashion. *SIDA*, then, is always already *sida*, which could explain the overwhelming popularity of the latter spelling in France. At any rate, the present study is clearly about *sida*.

A critical reading of scientific, literary, or popular representations that have emerged from the AIDS crisis should not consist in sorting out facts from fictions, or separating the true from the false. Rather, it should focus on identifying which representations constitute a resistant signifying practice and which ones do not. This does not mean, of course, that AIDS criticism should somehow fall outside the discourses it criticizes. In fact, AIDS criticism is a crucial part of the overall AIDS culture we live in, but its purpose should always be to bring us one step closer to the end of the epidemic. The strategy of a group such as ACT UP, for instance, functions at several levels simultaneously, and its dramatic accomplishments, whether in France, in the United States, or elsewhere, are largely due to a systematic awareness and criticism of dominant AIDS representations. For ACT UP, reading AIDS is fighting AIDS. Indeed, this should be the guiding principle of all AIDS criticism, including the present study.

AIDS Representations

Many representations used in the Western world to conceptualize our knowledge of the epidemic in its early years were often recycled from the long history of health and disease. Some figures came from the nineteenth century and the advent of modern medicine, some from earlier times. AIDS was initially explained with the help of metaphors and corresponding narratives thought to be obsolete but whose power and resilience were simply underestimated. Plague metaphors and their medieval overtones allowed some to construct AIDS as divine retribution when and where it affected primarily gay men, thus calling for radical political solutions. Leprosy conjured up the image of the body on which one can read the marks of otherness, while suggesting the exclusion of a community from the rest of society. Such metaphors directly fueled early calls to quarantine people with AIDS. Cholera, with its images of unwholesome environments, seemed an appropriate metaphor to use when denouncing and shutting down places for promiscuous gay sex, such as bathhouses, which, in turn, came to represent metonymically the gay community itself as a cesspool of infection. Tuberculosis, the romantic disease, brought to the image of AIDS its association with certain artistic and hypersensitive temperaments, now coded words for gay men, of course. The list could go on.

Susan Sontag and Sander Gilman have proposed some useful studies of the construction of AIDS in terms of past diseases and epidemics.[5] Gilman's approach, focusing mostly on the syphilis model, is particularly interesting inasmuch as it exemplifies both the strengths and limits of such archeological explanations of AIDS. First, Gilman links the iconography of syphilis through the past five centuries with that of AIDS, which was initially constructed as a sexually transmitted disease (*Disease and Representation,* 248). To simplify, let's say that in both cases we are dealing with an infection connected with a type of sexual behavior perceived as illicit or immoral, such as homosexuality, adultery, promiscuity, or prostitution. Gilman also notices the link with melancholia, depression, or the romantic image of the corrupt city. Such notions, as we have discussed earlier, culminated during the nineteenth century and were centered around the bourgeois construction of sexuality and, especially, degeneracy, a rhetorical concept ostensibly rendered useless since Auschwitz.[6] The greatest strength of Gilman's study is to show that such concepts have indeed survived and are ready to be used once again. Yet, this is also why his work's relevance appears somewhat limited when it comes to reading AIDS.

Gilman does not see the recycling of archaic figures as an attempt to incorporate as quickly as possible a new and threatening phenomenon in a more familiar, more established structure of knowledge. Instead, he proposes the following hypothesis: "the 'taming' of syphilis and other related sexually transmitted diseases with the introduction of antibiotics in the 1940s left our culture with a series of images of the morally infected and infecting patients suffering a morally repugnant disease but without a sufficiently powerful disease with which to associate these images. . . . AIDS was the perfect disease for such associations" (258). The problem with this explanation is that it inscribes AIDS in a long series of diseases, or rather "a series of images." It denies the cultural and historical specificities of these images, hence reducing them to an essentialist same/other dichotomy of which each "new" disease would only be the latest embodiment. While Gilman's observations are truly useful for our understanding of the early rhetorical constructions of AIDS, his conclusion, however, poses a serious problem if the purpose of all AIDS criticism should be to contribute to the solution of the crisis. Gilman's idea of available, idle figures in search of an object seems to imply the inevitability of AIDS, which finds itself inscribed in a global explanatory narrative, a teleology. It appears, then, that a purely analogical-archeological approach to AIDS runs the risk of being co-opted in a way Gilman or Sontag had not necessarily foreseen.

Indeed, many narrative frames, most of them already in place, began to determine the AIDS epidemic from the outset, to the point of making AIDS itself a narrative. The first AIDS narrative is of course the causal history of the syndrome, that is, the detective story, the whodunnit whose hero is the doctor/detective on the trail of the killer virus. As Treichler writes, regarding AIDS research, "a . . . consensus . . . emerged that basic research should now relate directly to the hypothesis that a single virus was the 'culprit' responsible for AIDS" ("AIDS, Homophobia, and Biomedical Discourse," 55). Such cause-and-effect narrative structure, which few people have seriously questioned,[7] directly originates from the paradigm of nineteenth-century medicine. There is no doubt that the hegemony of the virological explanatory narrative prevented the serious exploration of other avenues in the fight against AIDS. In fact, directly echoing this first narrative is the narrative of "the cure" or "the vaccine" modeled on that of the magic bullet.[8] This teleological frame so thoroughly structured AIDS research that life-prolonging treatments of the opportunistic infections contracted by people with AIDS were largely neglected until PWAs (People [or Person] with AIDS) themselves started to demand them.[9]

The other main narrative of AIDS tells us the story of the virus—how it came from the depths of the Dark Continent, transited Haiti, arrived in the United States and, from there, started to infect the rest of the Western world thanks to homosexual men, those ubiquitous sex pirates. Some critics have noticed how this story, beginning with the African green monkey and ending with the heterosexual white bourgeois, reuses the narrative sequence of Darwinian evolution.[10] Here again, a preexisting, ideologically loaded frame, based mostly on fantasmatic projections of Africa and of male homosexuality, helped determine an entire area of epidemiological research. As Watney remarks: "Thus 'prosti- tutes,' 'Haitians,' 'gay men,' 'Africans,' 'drug addicts' and so on have to be related to one another via narrative fantasies which tell us much about the unconscious of professional journalism, and nothing about actual epidemiology."[11] One could add, of course, that "actual epidemiology," too, is determined by such fan- tasies to begin with, and that one would be hard-pressed to find a "pure" epi- demiology that would not be tainted by some kind of metaphorical discourse. At any rate, Watney's observation reminds us how, just as in the nineteenth- century discourse of degeneracy, the black, the prostitute, the homosexual, the addicted still embody the threat of atavism—and powerfully so if one considers how successful these theories were, and still are.

Starting with these basic narratives—the virus, the cure, the epidemic—one can observe several genres emanating from popular fictions. The wide variety of these genres is a strong testimony to the evocative power of HIV and AIDS. Whether medical, journalistic, or fictional, all these narratives have one com- mon goal: to impose meaning on what does not have any. What is truly at stake, then, is the struggle for the power to attribute meaning.[12] For Judith Williamson, the concept of the abject as developed by Julia Kristeva helps to explain the pre- dominance of horror and melodrama in dominant AIDS discourses.[13] We shall come back later to the figures of the HIV-positive person and the PWA as metonymic embodiments of the virus, and how these figures reuse that of the vampire. For now, Williamson's analysis helps us understand how such narra- tives—which Crimp likens to Roland Barthes's notion of bourgeois writing[14]— allow the political dimension of the epidemic to be conjured away. Beyond the specific genres of horror and melodrama, Williamson's comments could equally apply to other genres, such as detective stories, spy or international terrorism stories, and science fiction. She writes, "What is so significant here is the *teleol- ogy* of the language, the implication that the virus is a subject—albeit a primi- tive one—with intentionality" (73; original emphasis); and later, "Suffering be- comes a commodity isolated from any systemic cause: just as the *source* of any problem can be located in Horror discourse in the Monster, equally its *effects* can be drained of any social dimension and lumped onto the individual Victim" (75; original emphasis). Yet, the cause of the AIDS pandemic, that is, not the exis- tence of HIV but the fact that the virus resulted in such a huge world crisis, is precisely systemic.

Of course, epidemics are social phenomena by definition and have always been linked to systemic factors. But the singularity of AIDS resides in the fact that it has affected not one specific marginalized or vulnerable segment of the population but many of them at once. According to Watney, the narrative struc-

ture of AIDS is different from that of other diseases precisely because of external factors, namely the links with the communities in which it was first noticed.[15] There can be no reason other than political to explain why the pandemic
started and continues to develop within segments of the world population
which have been disempowered in one way or another—gay men, IV drug
users, prostitutes, prison inmates, women, Africans and other populations from
developing countries, and ethnic minorities in industrialized countries.[16] Contrary to the humanist cant currently prevailing in Western countries—"AIDS is
everybody's disease," "Anybody can get AIDS," and so on—the epidemic does
not affect all of us in the same way. If, biologically speaking, anybody can get
AIDS, not everybody will.[17] AIDS metaphors, along with the constant threat that
they might translate into acts, clearly contradict humanist discourse.

In *AIDS and Its Metaphors,* Susan Sontag writes, "Of course, one cannot think
without metaphors. But that does not mean that there aren't some metaphors we
might well abstain from or try to retire" (93). What she is referring to in this passage is mainly the military metaphor so commonly used in AIDS rhetoric of all
kinds. Watney, Jan Zita Grover, and others have rightly underscored the theoretical impossibility of Sontag's injunction.[18] Nevertheless, her text represents a
good basis from which to analyze what, in certain metaphors and narrative
structures, may entail physical violence. To what extent is she right when she
states: "The metaphors and myths, I was convinced, kill" (102)? Undoubtedly
the many metaphorical and narrative projections framing the social groups initially associated with AIDS—particularly gay men and Africans—have influ-
enced early medical research and delayed prevention campaigns. It has been
said many times before, but it should be said many times again: if AIDS had first
been observed in members of less marginalized social groups, the pandemic
would not be what it is today.[19]

Predictably, AIDS itself has become a metaphor. In France, computers suffer
from *le sida informatique* and trees from *le sida des arbres.* In an infamous edito-
rial, Louis Pauwels wrote about *le sida mental* affecting high school students
demonstrating against the planned reform of French universities.[20] Everything
that can be metaphorically likened to a failure of the immune system may then
be given the name *sida X* or *sida Y.* It is tempting to read the proliferation of such
metaphors as a consequence of the epidemic's duration. Yet, since they appeared
relatively early on, I would suggest instead that they contributed to what has
been called the normalization of AIDS, that is to say the tendency in Western
countries to see the disease no longer as a crisis but as a social fact—not unlike
the Cold War and nuclear proliferation in earlier decades.[21]

Just as it was with late-nineteenth-century constructions of male homosexuality, Jewishness, racial and colonial otherness, et cetera, what is at stake in metaphorical and narrative uses of AIDS is truly the cohesion of national communities and the reinforcement of borders (in the literal and metaphorical senses of the term).[22] From the outset of the crisis, the old narrative of the virus of foreign origin made a dramatic comeback.[23] The pandemic was explained by the unprecedented mobility of the world's populations in the late twentieth century, the alleged cosmopolitanism of gay men, and so on. The metaphorical power of all infectious diseases, especially if they are new, mysterious, and lethal, found itself multiplied in the case of AIDS. The very idea of mobility thus becomes suspect; communication with the outside becomes threatening. Eventually, the reinforcement of borders and stricter immigration laws appear to be logical responses to the epidemic. It should come as no surprise that the "AIDS years" have seen an increase in official as well as nonofficial xenophobia in Western countries.[24]

HIV, which is believed to destroy the immune system, allows the metaphor to be inscribed both in the immunological and virological frames of the disease.[25] In previous chapters, we discussed how these two fairly recent frames actually echo two ancient concepts of medicine, and have long been used to articulate metaphors, particularly political metaphors. While the metaphor of viral invasion coming from the outside justifies the closing of borders, that of the internal collapse of our defense system can translate into authoritarian measures inside the national community. It is easy to imagine that the combination of both could be quite potent. Sontag notices how Jean-Marie Le Pen's Front National abundantly used the metaphorical potential of AIDS to strengthen its ultra-Rightist positions.[26] In his essay "Du fascisme sanitaire," Patrick Tort analyzes in political terms the use of metaphors in the rhetoric of Dr. François Bachelot, who was in charge of health issues in the Front National.[27] Tort articulates the moment when metaphors cease to be just that and begin to demand specific responses to the AIDS crisis:

> The recourse can be formulated in a strong and supremely convincing way: the fundamentalist protection of health becomes, *without metaphors*, the central theme around which all acts of exclusion, elimination, and persecution are constructed and legitimated: isolation, regrouping, concentration, testing, control, rejection, purge. This is also why Dr. Bachelot has been accused by a huge section of the medical profession of expressing "scientific un-truths," and so he did: *in his shift from metaphor to reality, reality, for him, was only the realization of the metaphor.*

[Le recours peut alors se formuler de manière forte et souverainement convaincante: la protection intégriste de la santé devient, *sans métaphore*, le thème axial sur lequel se construit et se légitime toute procédure d'exclusion, d'élimination et de persécution: isolement, regroupement, concentration, dépistage, contrôle, refoulement, purge. C'est aussi pourquoi le Dr Bachelot a été accusé par une immense partie de la profession médicale d'émettre des "contre-vérités scientifiques," et il les a effectivement émises: *dans le passage entre la métaphore et la réalité, la réalité n'a été pour lui que la réalisation de la métaphore.* (44; my emphasis)]

That is precisely the underlying danger of metaphors in AIDS discourse, just as it is in anti-Semitic rhetoric: their shifting from fiction to reality, when rhetoric translates into actual violence against actual people. The rather predictable excesses of the far Right go far beyond the Front National, and only emphasize what is actually the central issue of metaphors in general: how, in the case of AIDS, they construct the meanings of AIDS, and infuse them into all branches of public discourse: journalistic, literary, biomedical, legal, et cetera.[28]

AIDS, then, appears to be profoundly connected to social order. If the idea of a direct relationship between disease and social disorder was systematically developed in the nineteenth century with the concept of public health, one century, two world wars and a few genocides later, it is still ready to use. Military metaphors, whether in the context of AIDS or not, are frequently used in public discourse because they tend to create a consensus, a *union sacrée,* or, more cynically put, they allow all opposition to be silenced, very much like what happens in a time of actual war. Whether the war is being waged on drugs, poverty, or any other social problem, the idea is that the nation should stand as one to fight the peril. The AIDS crisis, structured by metaphors and narratives waiting to be realized, may appear to be the consequence of a combination of several social ills—the dissolution of the family, the sexual liberation of the 1960s and 1970s, homosexual promiscuity, immigration, drugs, and so on—as well as to provide the golden opportunity for a vigorous return to social order. However, if we admit that on the one hand it is impossible to rid AIDS discourse of its metaphors, and on the other that these metaphors always contain the potential to be realized in actual political acts, the most effective strategy, then, may be to recuperate inevitable language constructs and turn them against the (symbolic, social, political) order that produced them.

As I discussed in the previous chapter, for that order—or any order for that matter—to survive, it must be framed by a set of borders.[29] These borders may very well be literal ones if the order we're dealing with is a nation. But, more interestingly, they are also the lines or bars articulating a long series of structuring dichotomies metaphorically summarized since the nineteenth century by the healthy/ill dichotomy. Treichler proposes a long list beginning with "self and not self, the one and the other, homosexual and heterosexual," ("AIDS, Homophobia, and Biomedical Discourse," 63–64). According to Williamson, who bases her analysis on Kristeva's notion of the abject: "what seems to be particularly frightening about AIDS is that it is linked to the *breakdown* of boundaries. The virus threatens to cross over that border between Other and Self: the threat it poses is not only one of disease but one of dissolution, the contamination of categories" (78; original emphasis). First of all, this type of threat is not limited to AIDS but can be observed in several other cases—in particular, transmissible diseases and diseases that disfigure or induce madness, that is, that brand you as Other. Whoever enters the parallel universe of disease has crossed a border. Second, the "contamination of categories" on which social order rests is not specific to AIDS either, but rather sends us back to the medical construction of homosexuality. Williamson seems to be aware of that link when she writes: "Gay and lesbian sex are not frightening merely because they are perceived as 'Other' but precisely because they suggest, or recall, the dissolution of binary categories on which straight-dom rests" (78). As we can see, neither one of these two notions is really new. What is, however, is their association in such a dramatic way. The figure of the person with AIDS has simply inherited all the metaphorical history of the modern homosexual to become *the* central figure of AIDS representations.

Constructing the AIDS Sufferer

The immediate and extraordinary success of the "homosexual explanation" of AIDS can be attributed to the staying power, more than one hundred years after its birth, of the homosexual type constructed by legal and biomedical discourses. From this perspective, the history of AIDS reads like the mere chronicle of a death foretold, the inevitable outcome prophesied by the narrative of degeneracy, the pathological destiny of the homosexual finally realized, only this time at the level of the entire group at the same time. In *Policing Desire*, Watney notices this reinscription of homosexuality in the medical register: "At this point the categories of health and sickness . . . meet with those of sex, and the image of homosexuality is re-inscribed with connotations of contagion and disease, a subject for medical attention and medical authority" (126). Hence the cruel paradox that governs the relationship between a gay man with HIV or AIDS and the doctor he needs but for whom he feels a historical distrust. Early on in the epidemic, in "Living with Kaposi's," Michael Lynch described this paradox of AIDS: "Like helpless mice we have peremptorily, almost inexplicably, relinquished the one power we so long fought for . . . : the power to determine our own identity. And to whom have we relinquished it? The very authority we wrested it from in a struggle that occupied us for more than a hundred years: the medical profession."[30]

Early AIDS critics and activists asked themselves how they could expect doctors and researchers to "find a cure" for AIDS. As we have discussed earlier in this book, since medicine acquired the powerful status of science, the health/disease dichotomy has become one of the prevailing metaphors for such boundaries between an ordered inside (the symbolic and social structure) and an abjected outside (what needs to be defined as Other and expelled for the structure to exist). Today, the AIDS crisis, affecting primarily categories of people already constructed as diseased, has entailed a brutal reinforcement of the metaphor and, in some corners of the medical establishment, of the doctor's function as border guard between inside and outside, health and disease.

Logically then, as the dominant discourses of AIDS reappropriate the nineteenth-century conflation of otherness and disease, they also look for, that is, construct, markers of that otherness on the PWA's body. Once again, visible symptoms are supposed to reveal the patient's essential identity. In this respect, just as in the old discourse of *dégénérescence,* gay men are not the only ones to embody such fantasies. As Watney rightly observes: "The HIV virus has manifested itself in three constituencies which are already feared and marginalised in the West—blacks, intravenous drug-users, and gay men. The presence of AIDS in these groups is generally perceived not as accidental but as a symbolic extension of some imagined inner essence of being, manifesting itself as disease" (*Policing Desire,* 8). But once again the pathologized figure of the homosexual stands at the center of that discourse. For one thing, the gay community has been the first and hardest hit in the West, and despite all the "degaying" of AIDS that occurred in the 1990s it is still a very powerful association. In addition, the modern gay man is often seen as the perfect propagator of epidemics since he has been constructed as essentially cosmopolitan and an unstoppable border crosser—a literalization, in fact, of the old invert as pathological transgressor of all sorts of symbolic boundaries. Ultimately, many on the far Right of the political spectrum believe that all cases of HIV infection can be linked to homosexuality in one form or another, including husbands who are secretly bisexual, helpless drug addicts ready to engage in gay sex for money, participants in sex-

ual tourism, gay blood donors, et cetera. It is as if the virus came from homosexuality itself and the pandemic was the fault of a society so depraved that it
condoned the sexual extremes of the 1970s.

The gay PWA, then, has a story—a story ending in his horrible yet predictable
death. Indeed, since the late nineteenth century, medicine had warned us of this
fate, and Watney remarks: "older metaphors of sickness and contagion have
been all but replaced by a discourse of fatality, with AIDS widely regarded as a
syndrome of voluntary, deserved collective self-annihilation—the long-awaited,
and oft prophesied spectacle of the degenerates burning themselves out" (*Policing Desire*, 21). Again, how could medical science bring unmitigated hope when
it produced that story now validated by AIDS?

Consider the case of Rock Hudson. In a way he is the ideal protagonist of
the AIDS story, but that story also contains its own contradiction. In "Rock Hudson's Body," Richard Meyer writes: "the spectacular contrast of Rock Hudson's
two bodies—before/after, well/ill, 1950s/1980s, and, implicitly, hetero/homo-
sexual—provides the central trope for the conceptualization of his AIDS" (277).
In fact, one could carry Meyer's analysis further and posit that, in the West, AIDS
in general has been structured along the same type of nostalgic dichotomies.
And the very idea of a teleology, of a fatal progression from homosexuality to
AIDS, automatically implies much more than just that. To reuse Meyer's list of
dichotomies, we can notice that "after" was always latent in "before," like "ill" in
"well," the 1980s in the 1950s, and homosexuality (as expelled abject) in heterosexuality. Through these representations, we begin to see how a system that
blames the epidemic on those most affected, that is, those at the margins of that
system, could in fact be structurally responsible for it.

Another preexisting figure used in the construction of the PWA is that of the
vampire. After emphasizing the sexual dimension of gothic literature, Christopher Craft shows the symmetry between vampirism in Bram Stoker's *Dracula*
and the thrill of sexual inversion.[31] Once again homosexuality appears to be the
ideal signifier of the dissolution of boundaries. But if, as I noted in an earlier
chapter, the homosexual metonymically signifies all the fears contained in the
discourse of *dégénérescence,* his relationship with the most popular monster of
the late nineteenth century, the vampire, must be far-reaching.[32] For Richard
Dyer, the vampire and the (presumably closeted) homosexual both have something like a secret identity which only the trained observer can discover.[33] To this
I will add the logical parallelism between the vampire hunter and the doctor.
In both cases, the authority is derived from the ability to tell who "is" and who
"isn't." The vampire hunter, flanked by his loyal assistants, is like the gothic version of the doctor. Dyer does propose a positive, that is, anti-homophobic recu-

peration of the vampire theme, but remarks that AIDS might compromise such an attempt (58).

Surely, it is no coincidence that the figures of the vampire and vampirism were integrated into dominant AIDS discourses as soon as transmission of a virus through blood and semen was suspected. In the context of the AIDS crisis, the exchange of bodily fluids reinforces the image of sexual predator and the idea of contagion already linking the vampire and the homosexual. Through both intimate sexual contact and exchange of blood, the victim crosses the boundary separating him/her from the Other, the nonself, and in turn becomes infectious.[34] The HIV-positive person, then, becomes a creature not unlike the degenerate homosexual of a hundred years ago: monstrous, infectious, cunning, and able to seduce and kill in the same gesture. As for the gay PWA at the "terminal phase," his wasted body is like his own picture of Dorian Gray, the horrible revelation of his deeper truth.[35] Ellis Hanson summarizes the link between the figure of the vampire and those of the homosexual and the PWA as follows:

> When I speak of the vampire as the embodiment of evil sexuality, I speak of gay men and people with AIDS in the same breath. I am talking about the irrational fear of PWAs and gay men who "bite." I am talking about essentialist representations of gay men as vampiric: as sexually exotic, alien, unnatural, oral, anal, compulsive, violent, protean, polymorphic, polyvocal, polysemous, invisible, soulless, transient, superhumanly mobile, infectious, murderous, suicidal, and a threat to wife, children, home, and phallus. (325)

The list is quite thorough, and the metaphor is automatically followed by the corresponding metonymy that adds the final touch to the picture. For if we reread Hanson's list we notice that the characteristics attributed to people with HIV or AIDS almost directly echo the qualities attached to HIV itself. In other words, the person *with* the virus *is* the virus.

This metonymic shift corresponds, first, to a rather common need to put a face on the disease, or, in this case, on an invisible virus. But in the case of AIDS, unlike that of other diseases such as polio or muscular dystrophy, a poster child was not easy to come by. For a long time, nearly all images of PWAs were meant to be repulsive. Their goal was not to have viewers contribute money to help the sick, but to turn those who were healthy away from the behaviors that were sure to make them monstrous.[36] Second, the metaphor of the body politic, which allows and structures the rhetoric of disease studied in this book, easily entails the shift from the sickness to the sick when we are dealing with an infectious disease. Thus, in the case of a viral infection, the infected person runs the risk of becoming, metonymically, the virus itself. The "virus carrier" is never just that, especially since he/she does not get rid of the virus by infecting someone else— just as the vampire does not get rid of his vampirism when he bites his victim. Finally, the link, or rather the shift, from the "homosexual" to the "PWA" reinforces the metonymic shift from HIV-positive to HIV thanks to a century-old fantasy. If the "effects of HIV" so resemble those of homosexuality in the nineteenth-century medical imagination—wasting, weight-loss, the progressive dissolution of the self—the cause must logically be the same. HIV causes the collapse of the body's immune system and homosexuality that of the body politic.[37]

The metonymy has two major consequences: it justifies the exclusion of the sick, and it worsens the pandemic. When we are urged to avoid all contact with the virus, we are also urged to avoid all contact with infected people. The sick person, represented as the undead, to reuse Hanson's term, becomes what Watney calls "He-with-whom-identification-is-forbidden" (*Policing Desire*, 12, 22). It comes as no surprise to see that dominant representations of PWAs tend to reuse some elements still widely used to depict the "problems" of homosexuality: rejection and solitude. But the rejection of PWAs by their families and friends, although shown as cruel, is always presented as inherent to the PWA's condition. (Parents and relatives who face all sorts of dangers to welcome back home the prodigal son are the true heroes here. The PWA is only a pretext for the heroic construction of the heterosexual couple or the family.)[38]

In the field of representations, this construction of the PWA has had several consequences. The first is that PWAs who did not exhibit the expected signs of bodily decay remained invisible in the media for many years. In fact, throughout the 1980s, and despite the increasing life expectancy of people with HIV or AIDS, the typical images of PWAs corresponded to the very last months of the disease's evolution—and only if the disease was clearly identifiable by the "general public." Bernard Sellier, a photographer and volunteer for Aides, the largest French grassroots association for AIDS actions and prevention, himself a PWA, tells the following story: "Is it so unbearable not to look frightening? A young journalist I met recently was blaming me for 'my face,' which wasn't that of the proper PWA, and decided that there was no point in taking a picture of me, because I wasn't the true image of AIDS!" ["Est-il si insoutenable de me présenter sous un aspect qui ne fait pas peur? Un jeune journaliste, rencontré dernièrement, me reprochant 'ma tête' qui n'était pas celle d'un sidéen conforme, concluait de l'inutilité de me photographier, car je n'étais pas l'image du sida!"][39] The word *conforme* clearly implies that there already is a conceptual framework in place to predetermine the gaze projected on the sick. The fact that, of late, images of healthy-looking PWAs have become increasingly common changes very innocence, by the inexorable logic that governs all relational terms, suggests guilt" (99). The guilty/victim dichotomy functions as follows: If there is a victim, there must be some sort of perpetrator. Even victims of natural disasters look for people to blame. In the case of AIDS, if the "victim" is a person with HIV or AIDS, the culprit is also a person with HIV or AIDS who, one way or another, infected the former. Victimhood and guilt, therefore, are virtually indistinguishable; hence the need to bring the notion of "innocent victim" into the equation. And who might that be? Usually the "innocent victim" is hemophiliac or has contracted HIV through a blood transfusion or is a health professional accidentally infected while tending an AIDS patient. One of the reasons why the so-called tainted blood scandal (when French hemophiliacs were given blood products known to be contaminated) stirred such strong emotions in France is because the "victims" were children, fathers, and husbands. If so many countries are reluctant to authorize for everyone the emergency AIDS treatments available to health-care professionals, it is because the infected people in this case are considered more innocent than those who engage in certain irresponsible, and therefore punishable, behaviors.[44] Other "innocent victims" include babies born from HIV-positive mothers,[45] or people contaminated by a sexual partner who hid his/her HIV status.[46] In short, the "innocent victim" is s/he-with-whom-identification-is-possible.

The question I turn to in the next chapter is where to situate Hervé Guibert in this general context of the 1980s (when most of his novels are set) and early 1990s (when they were published). To what extent is he a product of that context? To what extent did he alter it? How did he reclaim phobic constructions of the PWA in order to disrupt the dominant narrativizations of AIDS?

5

⌐∞

AIDS and the Unraveling
of Modernity

The Example of Hervé Guibert

Hervé Guibert's AIDS novels, published between 1990 and 1992, were the first literary testimonies of their kind to enjoy a vast critical and commercial success in France. Many reasons have been put forward to explain why Guibert became such a cultural phenomenon. For some, a young, handsome, dying Hervé Guibert embodied something like a romantic ideal of creativity and early death. For others, he represented a long French literary tradition of first-person introspection in the face of illness and death. For most, whether they praised or condemned him for it, Guibert's contribution was to be found in what he had to say not about AIDS specifically but about universal human concerns with life, love, creation, and death. While recognizing his importance in increasing AIDS awareness in French society, the activists of ACT UP-Paris were prompt to criticize him for ignoring the social and political dimensions of the AIDS crisis, and, in effect, encouraging a universalizing reading of his work that could only be complicit with the epidemic. In the frontlines of the AIDS world, Guibert was often perceived as a self-centered, self-aggrandizing artist who was of no use in the fight against the epidemic. Hence, ACT UP argued, his immediate, and eminently suspect, canonization: If Guibert could be so easily recuperated by the system responsible for AIDS, it was because he was on the wrong side of the fight, on the side of the disease.

It is true that, with Hervé Guibert, we find ourselves on the side of disease, but, I contend, in a way that is akin to Genet's strategy of border crossing as analyzed in chapter 3. Reappropriating exclusionary figures, Guibert, too, was unapologetic about his sexuality, and he often depicted sex acts in a very explicit fashion that many found shocking. Guibert, in fact, was not one to present a harmless, middle-class image of gayness that had been sanitized for the public's protection—quite the contrary, as we shall see. Yet, like Genet before him, he was fully aware of the ambiguity of his position, that is, he was also operating within the very system that defined him as Other and sick. In what follows, I show that, although Guibert's strategy was not one of explicit political *engagement* or confrontational activism, his novels nonetheless propose a radical destabilization of the traditional health/disease rhetoric and the power structure that rests on it. My reading focuses particularly on Guibert's subversion of the medical gaze and the doctor-patient relationship; his redefinition of subjectivity, no longer in terms of the wholeness and health that had defined the modern subject, but rather in terms of disease; and his elaboration of a discourse that takes disease and contamination as the defining principles of language itself, and for which rumors and gossip may provide a discursive model.

Hervé Guibert

At the time he published his first novel dealing directly and primarily with AIDS, *A l'ami qui ne m'a pas sauvé la vie*, Hervé Guibert was a rather prolific albeit not widely read author. Since 1977 he had published many mostly autobiographical novels, as well as short stories, a screenplay, and essays.[1] He was also a photographer and photography critic for the daily newspaper *Le monde*. In the spring of 1990, when *A l'ami* was published, condom ads had been authorized and the first official prevention campaign had taken place only three years before. Aides, the association founded by Michel Foucault's longtime lover Daniel Defert after the death of the former, was not the huge organization it is today; ACT UP-Paris had come into existence less than a year before and was not yet known to the mainstream public. The only semi-celebrity who had declared publicly that he had AIDS was the essayist and journalist Jean-Paul Aron. And the few AIDS novels or testimonials that had come out were far from being best sellers. But on 16 March 1990, Guibert's TV appearance on the famous literary talk show *Apostrophes* made him an overnight media sensation. He had an extraordinary impact on the public. Although he looked obviously ill and tired, his youth and beauty may have had a lot to do with his success: in a sense Hervé Guibert became the face of AIDS in France.[2] *A l'ami*, a huge critical and commercial success, was followed in 1991 by *Le protocole compassionnel*, although Guibert had said that he would never write again. On 27 December 1991, he died shortly after a failed suicide attempt on the eve of his thirty-sixth birthday. A month after his death, his video-diary *La pudeur ou l'impudeur* finally aired on French TV. Several texts were published posthumously, including *Cytomégalovirus*, a brief diary of his hospitalization.

There is no question that Guibert had a tremendous influence on the general perception of AIDS in France, and particularly on media constructions of people living with HIV or AIDS. In the United States, such impact on the so-called general public is often achieved by the disclosure that an already famous person has HIV or AIDS. Rock Hudson was the first example, but there were also Magic Johnson, Arthur Ashe, and Greg Louganis, to name a few. In France, on the other hand, the phenomenon has been somewhat reversed, as some people became famous when, and because, they went public with their illness. In that sense, Guibert certainly started a kind of cultural trend. After him, Pascal de Duve also appeared on TV to promote his successful book, *Cargo vie*, and Cyril Collard became a huge star with the film adaptation of his earlier novel *Les nuits fauves*. All three were queer, and all three had an influence on the evolution of the PWA as a cultural construct. The question is, what kind of influence?

For ACT UP-Paris, Guibert and the others did not offer a genuine challenge to dominant representations of PWAs. Quite the contrary—they only reinforced stereotypes and capitalized on them for their personal construction as heroes. A new image of the PWA had simply been added to the old ones: "the HIV-positive artist staging his own seropositivity in a heroic light" ["le créateur séropositif qui met en scène sa séropositivité sous un aspect héroïque"].[3] Guibert, for one, claimed the hero label quite explicitly, as he told his interviewer on the TV show *Ex Libris:* "almost in the antiquated sense of the term, AIDS has made a kind of hero out of me . . . a character threatened . . . by death" ["le sida, un peu au sens vieillot du terme, a fait de moi un peu un héros . . . un personnage menacé . . . par la mort"].[4] If we read in "the antiquated sense of the term" a trace of irony rather than an uncritical reappropriation of traditional heroism, we could interpret Guibert's comment as an interesting twist on the (then) dominant images of the PWA as either victim or killer. While still framing his position in narrative terms, he would be subverting the dominant narrativization of AIDS by turning it against itself. But at the heart of ACT UP's criticism was the fact that Guibert and other young authors depicted their illness as a strictly individual adventure, thus presenting AIDS as the motor of a personal narrative rather than the result of a specific social and political context. Such depictions, ACT UP claims, can only worsen the AIDS crisis:

> Neither Hervé Guibert nor Cyril Collard engage in major reflections on the social origins of AIDS, or on the social conditions of its transmission. AIDS is an outrage for neither one of them. . . . : it is only about their personal destiny as an artist. They never set the problem in concrete terms, hardly even in medical terms, surely never in political terms. AIDS is destiny, it's fate, and therefore providence, redemption. . . . Whether fueled by compassion or by hatred, all teleological discourse on AIDS plays into the hands of the epidemic.

> [Ni Hervé Guibert, ni Cyril Collard ne se répandent en réflexions sur les origines sociales du sida, sur les conditions sociales de sa transmission. Ni pour l'un, ni pour l'autre, le sida n'est un scandale . . . . : il ne s'agit que de leur destin individuel de créateur. Jamais la question n'est posée en termes concrets, tout juste l'est-elle en termes médicaux, en tous cas jamais en termes politiques. Le sida, c'est le destin, la fatalité, et donc, la providence, la rédemption. . . . Qu'il soit compassionnel ou haineux, tout discours téléologique sur le sida fait le jeu de l'épidémie. (ACT UP-Paris, 176–77)]

In short, ACT UP sees the success of Guibert and others as fundamentally suspect since it has been used to reify new clichés and prevent the multiplicity of competing images: "It is indeed such quasi-unanimous success that is problematic. A univocal image of the PWA has been socially sanctioned as a result, in the absence of competing representations" ["C'est en effet ce succès quasi unanime qui fait problème. Une image univoque du séropositif s'en est trouvée socialement consacrée, en l'absence de représentations concurrentes"] (178–79). In *Sain[t]s et saufs*, Alain Ménil proposes a very similar interpretation of why Guibert and others were so successful. According to him,

> media exposure does not favor all works equally, for it also selects those that best lend themselves to a stereotypical and sensational approach. Again, why did the media focus their attention on Cyril Collard, Hervé Guibert, and Pascal de Duve, rather than others? . . . because their work did not disturb in any way the preexisting framework of disease representations.

> [la médiatisation ne profite pas identiquement aux oeuvres, car elle sélectionne aussi celles qui se prêtent le mieux à l'approche spectaculaire et stéréotypée. Là encore, pourquoi l'attention des médias a-t-elle retenu

Cyril Collard, Hervé Guibert ou Pascal de Duve, plutôt que d'autres? . . . car leur oeuvre ne bouleversait en rien le cadre préétabli des représentations attachées à la maladie. (132)]

And he goes on to add that books such as Guibert's reinforce "the cliché of one's death being not only accepted but even secretly desired" ["le cliché de la mort librement acceptée, sinon secrètement recherchée"], which creates "an intimate complicity between the ill person and his/her illness" ["une intime complicité du malade avec sa maladie" (132)]. While very reductive, such reading of Guibert as a social phenomenon, that is, as an important part of the public discourse on AIDS in France, is also largely accurate. It is undeniable that Guibert's public image as a PWA has been efficiently co-opted and incorporated into an evolving but still normalizing knowledge of AIDS. Yet who, or what, is to blame for this? To what extent are Guibert's texts actually complicit in what is after all a predictable attempt from any hegemonic discourse to retain its power position? As I suggested at the beginning of this chapter, Guibert's complicity with dominant systems of representation must be understood as part of a much broader strategy of destabilization.[5]

At first glance, though, Guibert's novels and public comments seem to confirm his detractors' criticism by depicting a purely personal experience of AIDS and inscribing this experience in the global autobiographical narrative that structures and defines his entire work. There is the oft-quoted remark from *A l'ami:* "AIDS will have been a paradigm in my project of self-revelation and the expression of the unspeakable" (228; translation modified) ["le sida . . . aura été pour moi un paradigme dans mon projet de dévoilement de soi et de l'énoncé de l'indicible" (247)].[5] There are also the numerous comments made by Guibert in interviews, such as the following:

> If it hadn't been AIDS, it would have been another disease in old age or any other confrontation with death. This is my thirteenth book, and if it hadn't existed, I would have had a feeling of incompletion. This book is not a testament, but it provides keys to understanding what was in all the other books and that sometimes I couldn't understand myself. AIDS has allowed me to further radicalize certain narrative systems.

> [Si cela n'avait pas été le sida, cela aurait été une autre maladie dans le grand âge ou toute autre confrontation avec la mort. C'est mon treizième livre, et s'il avait dû ne pas exister, j'aurais eu le sentiment de quelque chose d'incomplet. Ce livre n'est pas un testament, mais c'est un livre qui donne des clés pour comprendre ce qu'il y avait dans tous les autres livres

In France, until the rise of ACT UP-Paris and the boom of the gay community since the early 1990s, AIDS had almost exclusively been constructed as a personal tragedy. For one thing, such individualization was seen by many as a condition of *dédramatisation,* and as strategically necessary to counter the collective scapegoating discourse of Le Pen's Front National. But it is also inscribed in certain cultural traditions.[13] In modern French culture, illness is generally considered a private matter, and AIDS, initially linked to sexuality, and homosexuality to boot, was considered even more private. Given all these reasons, the (auto)biographical narrative appears to be the most appropriate literary form for conveying the experience of French gay men living with AIDS.[14]

And again, Guibert's AIDS novels seem to fit that cultural model perfectly. They are written in the first person and depict the illness and subsequent self-discovery of the narrator, a young Parisian gay writer named Hervé Guibert. In *A l'ami qui ne m'a pas sauvé la vie,* Hervé also tells the story of the illness and death of his friend Muzil, a philosopher modeled after Guibert's real friend Michel Foucault. But it is mostly a story of betrayals: that of Marine (Isabelle Adjani in real life), the temperamental movie-star friend, falsely rumored to have AIDS, who doesn't keep her promise to help Hervé have his script produced; and that of Bill, for whom the novel is titled, who leads Hervé to believe that he will be injected with a new experimental vaccine. Along the way, Guibert fictionalizes the creation of the nonprofit organizations Aides and Arcat-Sida. Besides Foucault, Adjani, Daniel Defert (Stéphane in the text), and Jonas Salk (Melvil Mockney), many other characters are relatively easy to identify. The second novel, *Le protocole compassionnel,* focuses more sharply on the personal experience of AIDS by the narrator, who, once on the brink of death, is now taking the new drug ddI. The gossipy dimension of the first book is much less evident in the second one, as Guibert's narrative focus shifts to his relationships with his doctor and other health-care professionals. In both texts, the habitual Guibert reader can recognize a familiar cast of secondary characters who had already appeared in his previous works. They include Hervé's old grand-aunts Louise and Suzanne; his lover Jules and the latter's companion Berthe, as well as the couple's two children; and Vincent, a straight occasional boyfriend. (There is also a third AIDS novel, *L'homme au chapeau rouge,* published posthumously, which I do not discuss here, as well as a short diary entitled *Cytomégalovirus,* written by Guibert during a hospital stay and also published posthumously.) To a large extent, all these texts find their place in Guibert's whole body of work, in a way that seems to bring thematic cohesion to an oeuvre that has now come to a close.

Emphasizing the inscription of *A l'ami* in the French literary canon, David Wetsel observes: "In the tradition of Montaigne, the novel's protagonist comes to have a kind of grudging respect for his illness. AIDS affords him a 'perspective intelligente'" (99). It is indeed difficult to read Guibert without being reminded of other sick first-person textual subjects such as Montaigne or Proust's narrator in *A la recherche du temps perdu,* to name only the most canonical. But it would be both reductive and ideologically suspect to read such intertextual connections as proof that Guibert is something like the latest representative of a long literary tradition, though hardly anything more. For one thing, both Montaigne and Proust occupy, for various reasons, a privileged position in the parallel canon of homosexuality. It is not my purpose, here, to read Guibert intertextually. My purpose, rather, is to show that Guibert's aesthetic choice of the first-person narrative, so criticized by ACT UP and praised, for the same reasons, by most critics, is not incompatible with a project of nonhegemonic redefinition of subjectivity—quite the contrary.

Returning the Doctor's Gaze

As I mentioned earlier, Guibert was not only a writer, but also a photographer. He was acutely aware of the role played by the gaze in the modern construction of subjects and objects, just as he knew the inherent violence involved in such positioning. In his AIDS novels, the issue of the gaze takes on a prominent importance as it comes to represent the moment when the PWA not only is constructed as object, but also when he or she can resist such construction and destabilize the subject/object dichotomy itself.

One of the narrator's earliest concerns is to avoid the authority of his parents' gaze. Guibert's meanness toward his parents was nothing new in his work; it culminated in his 1986 text entitled simply *Mes parents.* But in the context of the AIDS crisis and its popular representations, there is much more at stake than settling a score. In fact, the construction of AIDS as a family crisis has become the basis for much of the compassionate, liberal discourse on the epidemic. The earliest example of this trend is probably *An Early Frost* (1985), the first commercial movie about AIDS—actually an American TV movie—which was very widely seen and well received internationally, including in France. In it, we see a white, middle-class family unite and fight bravely after having first solved the crisis triggered by the simultaneous confessions of the son/brother's homosexuality and of his illness with AIDS. Many others have followed with slight variations from the model. I am thinking of course of Jonathan Demme's 1993 film *Philadelphia,* but also Christopher Reeve's 1997 cable movie *In the Gloaming.*[15]

In his novels, Guibert clearly rejects what constituted at the time one of the very few images of AIDS (and homosexuality) considered acceptable by a large portion of the heterosexual public. At no point are the narrator's parents directly present in the story. They barely intervene at all, and when they do, it is either on the phone or as a memory. In other words, the parents' gaze is never directly cast on the narrator as a PWA. As a result Guibert resists his construction as repentant prodigal son and disrupts the simultaneous construction of the parents as heroes. For him, the parents' gaze plays a central role in the wider social construction of the sick person as object, a process he sees as fundamentally violent. Talking about his illness, the narrator explains:

> If I were to tell my parents, I'd risk having the whole world dump shit on my head, all at the same time, I'd be letting every last asshole on earth crap on me, letting myself be buried under their stinking shit. My chief concern, in this business, is to avoid dying in the spotlight of the parental eye. (*A l'ami*, 8)

> [L'avouer à mes parents, ce serait m'exposer à ce que le monde entier me chie au même moment sur la gueule, ce serait me faire chier sur la gueule par tous les minables de la terre, laisser ma gueule concasser par leur merde infecte. Mon souci principal, dans cette histoire, est de mourir à l'abri du regard de mes parents. (16)]

In the following novel, *Le protocole compassionnel,* the tone is slightly less aggressive, and Guibert's purpose is to avoid having his death co-opted by the heterosexual family frame described above. That would, in effect, give AIDS a redemptive value for past illicit behaviors, in this case homosexuality:

> This morning my mother was snivelling over the phone to me, I gave her a sharp ticking-off. She must be sensing my coming death, she cracked up. No, dear parents mine, you shall not receive my sick body, nor my corpse, nor my cash. I shall not come home to die in your arms as you hope, saying: "Papa—Maman—I love you". . . . You shall learn about my death from the newspapers. (42)

> [Ma mère m'a pleurniché dans l'oreille ce matin, je l'ai rabrouée. Elle devait sentir ma mort venir, elle a craqué. Non, mes chers parents, vous ne récupérerez ni mon corps malade, ni mon cadavre, ni mon fric. Je ne viendrai pas mourir dans vos bras comme vous l'espérez en disant: "Papa—Maman—je vous aime". . . . Vous apprendrez ma mort dans un journal. (53)][16]

Conversely, Muzil's family manages to keep control over the philosopher's body and shelter it from the outside to impose their own version of the cause of death. His sister has a page removed from the hospital's records so that no official mention of AIDS shall appear anywhere. In order for the PWA to maintain his integrity, Guibert tells us, the parental gaze must (and can) be avoided. When he writes that his parents will learn about his death in the press, he is suggesting that relocating his personal illness and death in the public sphere might, paradoxically, do the trick.

The medical gaze, on the other hand, cannot be countered so easily. For Guibert, the greatest violence is indeed that of the medical gaze which legitimates the subject/object relation and freezes it in the objectivity of medical discourse, a discourse constantly reinforced by the authority it enjoys far beyond the field of medicine.

After his first blood tests, the first intrusions of medicine within his body, the narrator finds himself entirely exposed to other people's gazes. Guibert accumulates scenes in which, for example, the narrator lies on an examination table, "humiliated, lying naked for more than an hour . . . on a chilly metal table under a skylight where I could be seen by some workmen up on the roof, unable to call anyone because they'd forgotten all about me" (A l'ami, 32–33) ["humilié, couché nu depuis plus d'une heure . . . sur une table de métal glacée, sous une verrière où pouvaient me voir des ouvriers qui travaillaient sur un toit, impuissant à appeler car on m'avait oublié" (41)]. In such scenes, nudity becomes the sign of the patient's humiliation and dehumanization. In a somewhat Foucauldian way, he notes: "I'd hurled my body into something that seemed to strip it of a will of its own" (A l'ami, 180) ["j'avais lancé mon corps dans quelque chose qui le dépossédait apparemment d'une volonté autonome" (198)]. From then on, resistance will take the simple and immediate form of symbolic acts, as in *Cytomégalovirus,* when Guibert refuses to wear "[t]he transparent blue gown [which] had no purpose other than humiliation" ["La blouse bleue transparente [qui] n'avait d'autre fonction que l'humiliation" (60)]. He walks down to the operating room wearing plain clothes and a hat, before putting on the same green gown the doctors wear. Such an act, the appropriation and resignification of the doctor's clothes, constitutes in itself an act of resistance insofar as it re-creates the symbolic construction of the "doctor" and, implicitly, of the "patient." By repeating and imitating such a construction, he denaturalizes these two categories, and directly confronts the power relationship that governs them.

This appropriation of the other's clothes, which mimics power and reduces it to a question of attire, recalls what Judith Butler writes about Harlem drag balls in Jennie Livingston's *Paris Is Burning:* "Drag is subversive to the extent that it reflects on the imitative structure by which hegemonic gender is itself produced and disputes heterosexuality's claim on naturalness and originality" (*Bodies That Matter,* 125). If Guibert cannot avoid the surgery, if he has no other choice than to enter into a relationship with a doctor, he can at least change the game and impose the rules of his own survival. Butler calls this type of resistance "the forcible approximation of a norm one never chooses, a norm that chooses us, but which we occupy, reverse, resignify to the extent that the norm fails to determine us completely" (126–27). Guibert repeatedly does this to resignify his relationship to his doctor.

But his first reaction to the medical gaze is one of refusal: the refusal to be photographed or weighed, the refusal to know his latest test results, the refusal to submit himself to useless and painful exams, and so on. From this first stage on, Guibert proposes competing self-portraits, in which his beauty seems to increase as his body decays:

> I saw myself at that moment in a mirror, and thought I looked extraordinarily handsome, when for months I'd been seeing nothing more in my reflection than a skeleton. I'd just discovered something: in the end, I would've had to get used to this cadaverous face that the mirror invariably shows me, as though it already belongs no longer to me but to my corpse, and I would've had to succeed, as the height or renunciation of narcissism, in loving it. (*A l'ami,* 223)

> [Je me suis vu à cet instant par hasard dans une glace, et je me suis trouvé extraordinairement beau, alors que je n'y voyais plus qu'un squelette depuis des mois. Je venais de découvrir quelque chose: il aurait fallu que je m'habitue à ce visage décharné que le miroir chaque fois me renvoie comme ne m'appartenant plus mais déjà à mon cadavre, et il aurait fallu, comble ou interruption du narcissisme, que je réussisse à l'aimer. (242)]

One day as the narrator, visibly very ill, is riding the bus, a passenger recognizes him and says she finds him very handsome. Moved to tears, the narrator thinks: "Yes, it was necessary to see beauty in the sick, in the dying. Until then I had not accepted such a thing" (*PC,* 98) ["Oui, il fallait trouver de la beauté aux malades, aux mourants. Je ne l'avais pas accepté jusque là" (115)]. This new and sudden awareness is immediately followed by the realization that the photograph of a dying Mapplethorpe on the front page of *Libération,* although shocking at first, is beautiful after all. When Guibert assumes the image of the AIDS patient with his decaying body to signify beauty, the act becomes a subversive reiteration. This beauty of the AIDS patient is not a beauty *despite* his illness, which would remain within the frame of humanistic yet exclusionary representations as in *Philadelphia;* rather it is a beauty *within* the illness.

Humanistic representations of both the patient and the doctor reiterate, in order to reinforce, the symbolic construction of subjects and objects. The so-called dignity of the dying, and especially of the "degenerate," whose horrible deaths constitute their mandatory redemption, consists in passively accepting exclusion and death as inevitable. With AIDS, more perhaps than with any other disease, to be beautiful in death would mean to assume the role of *pharmakos,* or scapegoat, and willingly embody otherness and death to protect the community. Guibert, however, does not let himself be passively looked at; he actively exposes himself. He keeps reminding the reader of how he refuses to let anyone take pictures of him, yet at that very time in the novel the narrator is also directing a video documentary about himself for television. In the narcissistic moment mentioned earlier, he simultaneously constructs himself as (desiring) subject and (desired) object, and he invites the reader to join in and watch.

At this stage, then, the reader looks in the mirror and sees the eroticized body of Hervé Guibert. The subject finds itself (re)constructed as a dying subject. Later, the narrator starts bringing his camcorder during medical exams or massage sessions, where the recorder on its tripod systematically reproduces the same mirror effect. Soon, the camcorder will mediate every description in the text of the narrator's body and nudity. As in the case of the mirror, the reader does not watch the scene directly, but instead watches it through a video camera set up by the narrator-patient who determines and mediates every outside gaze. Appropriating the very technology so widely used to construct the "AIDS patient," the narrator now uses that medium to contest his position as an object by exposing it as a construct. Nudity ceases to be the sign of humiliation. Instead, these scenes are the inverse of the earlier violent scenes in which the reader-voyeur found him- or herself in the position of the workers on the roof watching the forsaken body of the narrator.

The most unbearable and violent scene that Guibert describes is the fibroscopy in *Le protocole compassionnel,* in which the reader's gaze, this time, is not mediated. In this particular scene, the reader's position is that of the doctor "built like some Nazi sadist from the movies" (47) ["[au] physique de sadique de film de nazis" (58)] who directs his assistant during the operation, and gazes "through the eyepiece, from a distance" (47; translation modified) ["à l'oeilleton, à distance" (59)] to diagnose ulcers in the patient's stomach. Generally, Guibert's most violent scenes force the reader to occupy the place of the doctor (or the worker on the roof or a sadistic Nazi, et cetera) placing him or her in a position that, uncomfortable as it may be, allows the reader to become aware of the violence of a gaze that constructs the patient as "an auschwitzian panning" (6; translation modified) ["en panoramique auschwitzien" (14)].

In "Fantom Images," Emily Apter notes that Guibert "identifies the subversive homologies between sexual violation, nosological voyeurism, and the medical rape of the subject as crucial constituents of *sida* narrative" (84). Indeed, the violence of the fiberoptic exam finds a direct echo in the passage where the narrator is raped by Djanlouka, a straight teenager who tells the narrator that "he wanted to defy death. He had come for that purpose. He had brought a condom" (*PC*, 139) ["il voulait risquer la mort. Il était venu pour cela. Il avait apporté une capote" (163)]. This precaution suggests that the peril of death that so thrills Djanlouka resides less in the contact with the virus than in the homosexual act itself.

The violence to which PWAs are often subjected appears to be less an inherent aspect of "*sida* narratives" than a logical extension of medicalized homophobia. Such violence illustrates how the homosexual body represents a place where the heterosexual subject projects his morbid fantasies in a violent process of domination.[17] In the case of the fiberoptic exam, Guibert explains the brutality he felt during the procedure: "To Dr. Domer, I was nothing more than just another infected little faggot, who was going to kick the bucket in any case, and who was wasting his time" (47) ["Pour le docteur Domer, je n'étais qu'un petit pédé infecté de plus, qui allait de toute façon crever, et qui lui faisait perdre son temps" (58)]. In both cases, we are confronted with a violence that is legitimated in part by a modernized version of the century-old medical discourse that constructs the homosexual as a naturally diseased object and homosexuality as an abjected space of nonbeing. The violence becomes subsequently justified and multiplied by the juxtaposition of homosexuality and a lethal disease.

After the description of the fiberoptic exam, Guibert begins to propose a competing image of the patient, an image produced this time by the patient himself. This new image, however, does not constitute the "truth" of the patient; Guibert never claims to present such truths. Instead he actually exposes both the patient and the doctor as mere roles, produced by and in a discourse that claims to represent them objectively. Guibert, describing the pleasure he feels in appropriating the medical jargon, compares it to his own infectious blood—and invites his readers to share his blood:

> I like their fluid, almost natural speech, and now I like carrying my blood whereas before I'd have passed out, I'd have felt my knees giving way. I like there to be a direct line between my thought and yours, so that the style doesn't get in the way of the transfusion. Can you stand a story with so much blood in it? Does it turn you on? (*PC*, 89; translation modified)

[J'aime le langage fluide, presque parlé, et j'aime maintenant porter mon sang alors qu'auparavant je serais tombé dans les pommes, j'aurais eu les genoux coupés. J'aime que ça passe le plus directement possible entre ma pensée et la vôtre, que le style n'empêche pas la transfusion. Est-ce que vous supportez un récit avec tant de sang? Est-ce que ça vous excite? (105)]

In the context of AIDS, the words *fluide, sang,* and *transfusion* directly conjure up the idea of contamination. In this particular passage, the reader participates in this contamination by the very act of reading.

In the passage, Guibert gives the reader the opportunity to refuse to model his or her gaze after the doctor's at the same time that he forces the reader to adopt the point of view of a gay man with AIDS. Thus, like HIV, the text becomes a factor in the contamination of the reader—with the latter's assent. Moreover, in *Le protocole compassionnel,* written after the wide success of *A l'ami,* Guibert was perfectly aware of his larger and more diverse readership, which now included women and heterosexual men who, for the most part, had never read his books before.

Guibert, then, resists victimization by forcing his healthy, heterosexual readers to look through the eyes of someone who is ill, gay, and more. It is clear that Guibert does not seek to propose a sanitized image of homosexuality or AIDS. Instead he reiterates its most traditionally abject figures. He does not hide his taste for rough sex and S/M or his attraction for young boys, regretting only that the overall fear of sex he experiences as a result of his illness keeps him unable to carry out his desires: "The skeleton I have become apparently does not have the courage to warm himself with young boys, and feels very badly about it all" (*PC,* 73) ["Le squelette que je suis devenu n'a pas le courage apparemment de se réchauffer aux jeunes garçons, et il n'en est pas fier du tout" (89)]. Elsewhere, he compares himself to a child killer awaiting execution (63 [77]). He also presents with understanding sympathy Thierry Paulin, a gay man with AIDS who murdered several old women in Paris in the mid-1980s, and simply comments: "His serial murders were his own race against death" (77) ["Sa série de meurtres était sa course à lui contre la mort" (93)], thus establishing a disturbing parallelism between writing and serial killing. Guibert even reclaims the figure of the vampire, which, as we discussed earlier, has played a crucial role in the dominant construction of AIDS: "I take more and more pleasure in watching a fine fat vein in the handsome arm of a handsome boy being pierced by a needle. . . . Indeed, I'd like to take blood samples myself" (190; translation modified) ["J'aime de plus en plus voir une belle veine bien saillante d'un beau bras d'un beau garçon percée par une aiguille. . . . En fait, j'aimerais faire moi-même des prises de sang" (218)].

To complete his image of sexual predator, he adds:

> I have so little flesh now on my own bones . . . and I could easily become
> a cannibal. When I see the beautiful bare fleshy body of a worker on a con-
> struction site, I have a yearning not just to lick it all over, but to bite it, to
> batten on it, to gnaw it, to masticate it, to swallow it. . . . I would like to
> eat the raw, vibrant flesh, warm, sweet and filthy. (74; translation modi-
> fied)

> [Je manque tellement de chair . . . que je deviendrais volontiers cannibale.
> Quand je vois le beau corps dénudé charnu d'un ouvrier sur un chantier,
> je n'aurais pas seulement envie de lécher, mais de mordre, de bouffer, de
> croquer, de mastiquer, d'avaler . . . je voudrais manger la chair crue et vi-
> brante, chaude, douce et infecte. (90)]

The autonomy and cohesion of the healthy and heterosexual readers are threatened by the irruption not only of homosexuality and AIDS, but also pedophilia,
murder, vampirism, and cannibalism. Confronted with the possibility (indeed,
the inevitability) of being recuperated by a mainstream audience and assimilated into liberal, humanistic discourses, Guibert, not unlike Jean Genet before
him, reclaims and assumes radical difference. Such a strategy not only prevents
easy assimilation but also brings out the violence with which society regulates
and outlaws certain practices. Guibert makes it clear that he is not fighting for
acceptance and tolerance. If he does gain respect, it will be on his own terms.

Understandably, many readers may be reluctant to let themselves be exposed
to and manipulated by what they have heretofore repelled. The narrator, for instance, considers posing nude for a series of paintings titled *Nude suffering from
AIDS* (*PC*, 16) [*Nu malade du sida* (25)]. He also negotiates with a theater direc-
tor to appear nude on stage during the popular Avignon festival. But the latter
refuses: "'People will say,' he had said, 'that you are exposing yourself'" (16;
translation modified) ["On va dire, avait-il dit, que vous vous exhibez" (26)].
Even more telling is the decision of the TF1 television station to postpone
broadcast of the author's film. Why did TF1 executives refuse to broadcast, as
long as Guibert was alive, a film they had themselves commissioned and fi-
nanced? What is it about this film that made it "unshowable" before its creator's
death? In an interview given shortly before he died, Guibert himself noted: "Every channel refused. There must be something frightening about these images!"
["Toutes les chaînes ont dit non. Il faut croire que ces images font peur"].[18]

Indeed, if shown when Guibert was still alive, these images would have
threatened the hegemony of conventional media representations, which typi-

cally favors the figure of the passive, silent victim—such that these images would have benefited from the mass appeal of television. But what made the broadcasting of these resistant images so problematic in the eyes of television executives was that they confronted and exposed the role of the media in producing conventional representations and therefore in spreading the epidemic. That the film was not shown until after Guibert's highly publicized death seems to unveil an unrelenting teleology of redemption, and to give the audience the choice to see in the film a pathetic and useless fight against fate—a tragedy. Such an interpretation may not be the only one, but it is at least made possible, and even encouraged, by the context of the broadcast. The film could become a natural yet harmless tribute to the great departed writer. The history of AIDS is full of such acts of cowardice.

In *Le protocole compassionnel,* the taping of the film plays a double role. On the one hand, as we have seen, it allows Guibert to affect the reader's point of view by reproducing in the text the narcissistic gaze of the narrator. On the other hand, it deeply modifies the relation between doctor and patient by inserting the possibility of a second, competing gaze, that of the patient onto the doctor. The appearance of the camcorder in the doctor's office is going to disrupt a relationship previously based on the nonreciprocity of the medical gaze. Like photography in the nineteenth century, video has extended and reinforced the scientific gaze with the perceived objectivity of technology and the massive reproduction of new images. But today this production of so-called objective knowledge can be disseminated at a speed and in proportions that were unthinkable one hundred years ago. As a result, medical knowledge tends to become increasingly uniform. This, along with the power that has been ascribed to medicine, impedes the production of counterdiscourses on health and disease in general, and postpones the resolution of AIDS, the disease of the disempowered, in particular.

Wondering what he should or should not show in his movie, Guibert quickly abandons the idea of videotaping "these walking corpses" of other PWAs (*PC,* 36; translation modified) ["des cadavres ambulants" (46)], that is, of modeling his gaze after that of dominant TV-style documentary makers. Instead, the film soon adopts the fictional mode of the book itself. The first scene taped by the narrator is a massage session in which he divides himself in two in order to describe his own body from the point of view of the camera: "me, stark naked, I am filming this raddled nudity" (*PC,* 83; translation modified) ["moi nu comme un ver, je filme cette nudité décharnée" (99)]. "Me" as object of the gaze and "I" as subject come to occupy two different spatial positions. From this moment on, the scene is entirely described from the point of view of the camera, and the

movement of bodies as they will appear on screen. In lieu of a realistic effect
which would give the film the naturalizing look of a documentary, the *mise en
abyme* problematizes the representation of the medical act by adding an extra
level. Hervé Guibert becomes a character in the movie shot by Hervé Guibert,
the narrator of the novel written by Hervé Guibert.

But this doubling up goes even further, and implies the possibility of infinitely repeating the process. Truth, therefore, finds itself indefinitely post-
poned, while disease is exposed as a construct and the doctor is presented first
as some kind of literary critic and ultimately as a fictional character. "Doctor"
and "patient" cease to function as natural and clearly bounded identities, and
once again appear to be scripted roles: "On the work of the masseur and our
common labor is superimposed or underimposed the work of the film being shot, the filming of the two actors we most certainly are, actors blessed with
genius" (*PC,* 83; translation modified) ["Au travail du masseur et à notre
labeur commun se superpose ou se sous-perpose le travail du film en train de
se tourner, et dont nous sommes indéniablement les deux acteurs, des acteurs
pleins de génie" (99)]. The artificiality of both the masseur's and the patient's positions is reinforced by the term *sous-perpose,* which suggests that the work of
fiction does not complement but rather undermines them. The interference of
the camera, that is, of the patient's gaze onto the medical *scène* (both "scene" and
"stage") immediately delegitimates the traditional doctor-patient relationship,
exposes it as role playing, and opens up for negotiation everything that previously rested on such roles: knowledge, power, discourse, ethics, and the position they assign to the human body.

Claudette Dumouchel, the narrator's physician, immediately refuses to let
him videotape her during medical exams. Apter writes, "A private person dedicated to the confidentiality of her métier, Claudette refuses to be a party to such
exhibitionism" (94–95). But Dumouchel's refusal to appear on screen, as an image, may also have systemic rather than just personal causes. It constitutes a reluctance on her part to find herself "objectivized" by the patient's gaze, which
would reverse the implied hierarchy governing their relationship. The distribution of their bodies on the screen seems to entail more than the simple reversal
of placing the patient in the dominant position formerly occupied by the doctor. If indeed the doctor were to lose her position of power by letting herself be
videotaped, she would also be forced to acknowledge the fact that the video not
only represents such a position but actually produces it. The camera's gaze
would be simultaneously and evenly cast on both herself and the patient, thus
denaturalizing their respective identities. The following conversation between
doctor and patient suggests that the doctor cannot accept the idea that her po-

sition of power depends only on the discourse that produces it as such: "'But after all you can't very well prevent me from filming, it's my body, it's not yours.' 'Yes,' said Claudette, 'but my own body would be forced to enter the frame in order to examine you'" (*PC*, 197; translation modified) ["Vous ne pouvez tout de même pas m'empêcher de me filmer, c'est mon corps, ce n'est pas le vôtre.— Oui, répond Claudette, mais mon corps à moi sera bien forcé d'entrer dans l'image pour vous examiner" (225)]. According to Apter: "In a sense, both are arguing that some breach in the ethics of medical distance is inevitable with this kind of illness" (95). Again, it seems that Guibert goes far beyond adapting professional ethics to fit a new disease. The presence of the camera alters the relationship in a fundamental way.

When he films, Guibert is theoretically on both sides of the camera, as he and the doctor appear simultaneously on screen. The situation has two immediate consequences: first, the patient's position both behind and in front of the camera prevents him from simply occupying the unified authoritarian subject position previously occupied by the doctor; second, the doctor's presence on the screen alongside her patient levels their relationship. The doctor, too, has a body, and, for a change, it is hers and not the patient's which is "forced to enter the frame." What do we have, then? On the one hand, there is the absence of the subject, because there really is no one physically behind the camera; on the other, there is a doctor reduced to a role determined by the patient who stages her relationship to him. In both cases, the kind of subjectivity embodied in the traditional doctor-patient relationship finds itself weakened and its naturalness radically negated, as the empty space behind the camera visualizes the notion that the subject is only a position constructed by a system of representation.

In this instance, Guibert's politics seem to be much closer to ACT UP's than some would have it. Consider, for example, how Philippe Mangeot, president of ACT UP-Paris and one of Guibert's most vocal critics, defines the subversive dimension of AIDS activism:

> The ACT UP experience is subversive where it opens up breaches, like within the rules governing political transaction or in the mastery of medical knowledge. . . . When we slip into the role of the expert, when we acquire his knowledge, but reclaim that knowledge from our position as patients, whereas the expert is supposed to abstract himself from his object and study it in a neutral fashion, then we subvert the very identity of the expert: Nobody ever is in his or her place when dealing with an interlocutor who claims to occupy two positions at once, in this case that of the expert and that of the patient.

[L'expérience d'Act Up est subversive là où elle ouvre des brèches, par exemple dans les règles de la transaction politique ou dans la maîtrise du savoir médical. . . . Quand nous nous glissons dans le rôle de l'expert, que nous acquérons son savoir mais que nous revendiquons ce savoir depuis notre place de malade, alors que l'expert est sensé [sic] s'extraire de son objet et prétend l'aborder avec neutralité, nous subvertissons jusqu'à l'identité même de l'expert: personne ne peut plus être vraiment à sa place quand, en face de lui, il a un interlocuteur qui prétend occuper deux places à la fois, en l'occurrence celle de l'expert et celle du malade.][19]

This is in essence what Guibert does in *Le protocole compassionnel*.

But the eroticization of the Guibert-Dumouchel relationship complicates things even further. Much has been written about the history of women being eroticized through the gaze (and subsequent work) of male painters, photographers, and filmmakers.[20] Might Dumouchel's initial reluctance to be videotaped reflect a refusal as a woman—not as a doctor—to see her image fixed once again by the male gaze? The very notion of a hierarchized and authoritarian relation between subject and object has been disrupted, and not merely displaced, by the patient's resistance. The erotic dimension of Guibert and Dumouchel's relation does not aim at heterosexualizing the male narrator at the expense of the female doctor. Rather it shows the interdependence of their positions within the discourse which produces them.

The "You-Me" exercise (designed to test the sensitivity of the patient's toes) becomes an erotic pendulum-like movement between doctor and patient:

Now she is holding my big toe, and I have to tell her if she is bending it up or down, towards her or towards me. My eyes remain closed, she manipulates my big toe and I have to say: "You. Me. You. You. Me. Me. You. Me. You. You. Me." I keep saying me-you, me and you, until I start panting, out of breath. (*PC*, 37)

[Maintenant elle prend mon gros orteil, et je dois dire si elle le positionne en arrière ou en avant, c'est-à-dire vers elle ou vers moi. J'ai les yeux fermés, elle bouge mon doigt de pied et moi je dis: "Vous. Moi. Vous. Vous. Moi. Moi. Vous. Moi. Vous. Vous. Moi." Je lui dis moi-vous, moi et vous, jusqu'à bout de souffle, jusqu'à en perdre haleine. (47)]

And the boundaries become all the more blurry when Guibert says "We're playing doctors" (*PC*, 37) ["On joue au médecin" (47)]. In this sense, the game of "You-Me" has the same denaturalizing effect as the "actors'" performances in the film. And later Guibert writes: "I undress, and I get in the picture. Claudette joins me" (*PC*, 198; translation modified) ["je me déshabille, et j'entre dans l'image. Claudette m'y rejoint" (226)].

Thus, the picture ceases to be the frame which fixes the identities of both the patient and the woman as objects. Instead, it becomes the open space of a dynamic love relationship, destabilizing identities and exposing them as constructs. It is clear, however, that heterosexuality, while the narrator toys with an idea so new to him, remains this "something else altogether that I shall never know" (*PC*, 90–91; translation modified) ["autre chose que je ne saurais jamais" (107)]. The eroticization of his rapport with Claudette Dumouchel never translates into a reconstruction of traditional male subject and female object positions, as if to compensate for the unbalanced doctor-patient relationship. If that were the case, the notion of subject and object as natural categories and the principle of domination that structures it would not be questioned but only displaced laterally and embodied by two other but equivalent hierarchized dichotomies: male/female and hetero/homo.

On the contrary, Guibert explicitly evokes the sadomasochistic dimension of his relation to Dumouchel, a dimension that directly echoes his homosexuality as presented in his earlier writing. Moreover, he is the one occupying the "passive" role, as shown by their respective positions during medical exams but also through various puns such as "Waiting for Claudette to take me" (*PC*, 196; translation modified) ["En attendant que Claudette me prenne" (224)]. Mainly, the analogy of sadomasochistic sex, an extremely codified game of role-playing and itself a staging of power relations, reinforces the idea that the doctor-patient relationship takes place on a stage where roles may be forever interchangeable. After all, "We're playing doctors."

From the recognition of this role-playing arises the possibility of constructing a new patient-doctor relationship on a different basis, one that now acknowledges the mutual dependence of the two positions—the abjected outside being constitutive of the inside—and the absence of hierarchy between them. As Guibert writes: "The doctor along with his patient have to invent a healing relationship" (*PC*, 68; translation modified) ["Le médecin et son malade doivent inventer ensemble la relation bienfaisante" (81)], which implies that the relation must be the result of a negotiation. Here Guibert seems to suggest that such negotiation could elaborate medical knowledge both within and through the patient-doctor relationship. He mentions the example of a successful alveolar cleansing "despite the barbarity of the act itself" because it became "almost a quartet in which I was the fourth voice playing with the complicity of the other three" (*PC*, 62; translation modified) ["malgré la barbarie de l'acte lui-même [parce qu'il] devint presque un quatuor dont je jouais la quatrième voix avec la complicité des trois autres" (*PC,* 75)]. The patient's "voice" becomes an integral part of the process, which was not the case during the earlier, extremely brutal fiberoptic exam. Later, Guibert writes about his nascent relationship with Dumouchel: "the relationship must be allowed to build up all on its own using looks and words, the two of us, speaking openly, together. We have to go on inventing it" (*PC,* 87; translation modified) ["il faut laisser la relation se bâtir toute seule sur les regards et les paroles, à deux, de vive voix, ensemble. Il faut continuer de l'inventer" (103)]. The patient-doctor relationship is a dynamic process, constantly being invented, and not a fixed, preexisting model. Guibert has overcome the tactical phase of refusal, the refusal of the automatic status of the patient, the refusal of the doctor's knowledge and power, to enter the stage of negotiation and elaboration of a new, nonhegemonic type of subjectivity.

The Diseased Subject

The next question is: What kind of subject can emerge from this newly redefined relationship if we are not dealing with a mere inversion of value between binary opposites? I suggested that the intrusion of the camera prevented the repositioning of the patient as a full, homogeneous subject, and therefore the reinforcement of hierarchized dichotomies. In "The Mirror and the Tank," Lee Edelman uncovers the reconstitution of precisely such exclusionary dichotomies in the rhetoric of a certain type of AIDS "activism." Constructed as the opposite of "passivity" and "narcissism," two qualities traditionally associated with gay men, activist rhetoric reproduces the latter's exclusion. As an alternative practice, Edelman proposes "to reinvent ourselves and our social relations, insofar as that can be done, by trying to imagine new subjectivities whose pleasure and politics no longer require conceptualization through antithesis" (34). Based on the scene in *A l'ami* in which Guibert recognizes his own beauty in the mirror, Edelman stresses "the need to love, not leave, the mirror, by rediscovering the luxury of narcissism from within an experience constructed on every side as a rupture in narcissism itself" (33). In *Le protocole compassionnel,* perhaps even more than in *A l'ami,* Guibert allows us to envision a more radical fracture, constitutive of what I would term the diseased subject.

Logically, the doctor's office turns out to be the privileged locus for the elaboration of the diseased subject because its first strategic stage is that of the "diseased as subject." We already showed how the reciprocity of the gaze allowed Guibert to destabilize the institutionalized positions of both patient and doctor, and to suggest the inevitability of their inversion. What emerges from then on is the possibility of conceiving doctor and patient as two distinct yet mutually contaminated positions, internally fractured by the explicit and constant recognition of the other's constitutive presence in each one. In *Cytomégalovirus*, when the narrator refuses to wear the humiliating gown especially designed for patients, he tells the nurse: "The only way you could make me accept it would be for you to come down with me, hand in hand and wearing the same outfit" ["La seule façon pour vous de me le faire accepter serait que vous descendiez avec moi dans la même tenue, main dans la main" (58)]. Finally, as we saw earlier, he ends up wearing the same gown as the doctors during the operation. As the episode suggests, the faultline separating doctor and patient finds itself displaced, and now runs through each one rather than between them, thus preventing their full self-presence and plenitude as subjects.

The diseased subject also experiences its fracture by reclaiming, this time, its loss of selfhood. In *A l'ami*, the narrator recounts the initial loss of identity suffered by himself and Muzil and to which everyone is subjected as soon as he or she is assigned the identity of "patient." Little by little, however, that very loss of identity is resignified positively as the patient becomes a member of a community. In the case of AIDS the assignation of PWAs to one community or another is always implied by dominant discourses—even negatively, as in "not gay." Membership is determined by the presumed cause of infection and the community gives both its coherence to the personal narrative of the "case history" and its identity to the protagonist of that narrative. Membership in a community must therefore be exclusive. Guibert, however, outlines a more complex network of relations.

In "Traces and Shadows," Ralph Sarkonak recognizes that Guibert's novels have a political dimension, but he sees it as a simple redefinition of the traditional notion of family. Guibert goes much further than that. At first, the narrator and his immediate circle of friends are presented as doomed: "We're all going to die of this disease, me, you, Jules, everyone we love" (*A l'ami*, 104) ["On va tous crever de cette maladie, moi, toi, Jules, tous ceux que nous aimons" (117)]. When a doctor denies Guibert the right to see Muzil alive one last time, it is because "blood relatives came first" (*A l'ami*, 93) ["la loi du sang . . . privilégiait les membres de la famille" (106)]. For Guibert, of course, being HIV-positive creates a different group of "blood relatives," a much stronger "loi du sang." But the limited universe of the inner circle is soon expanding as Guibert begins to depict the heterogeneous but increasingly solidary crowd at the hospital or the grassroots organization created by Muzil's lover Stéphane. And when Marine appears on TV to dispel the rumors of her death from AIDS, she says "she was distressed to be betraying those who were really sick, and to have to place herself publicly like that among the ranks of the healthy" (A l'ami, 117) ["elle était navrée de trahir le camp des malades, et de devoir s'afficher comme ça dans celui des bien-portants" (131)]. To be sure, Guibert is highly critical of Stéphane, Marine, and many others, but even so, his depictions allow him to go beyond AIDS as a strictly personal experience. In the following novel, the community of the sick, in its very diversity, actually becomes an essential part of that experience. Hence, as the diseased subject displaces yet another faultline—that between the PWAs themselves—self-identification becomes a plural process of relationships.

The fracture of the diseased subject, however, is most dramatically figured by the descriptions of the narrator's premature aging. A l'ami closes with the narrator's return to his childhood: "My muscles have melted away. At last my arms and legs are once again as slender as they were when I was a child" (246) ["Mes muscles ont fondu. J'ai enfin retrouvé mes jambes et mes bras d'enfant" (267)]. These are the very last words of what Guibert claimed at the time to be his very last novel. The reader is left to imagine the progressive dissolution of the subject toward nonbeing. But the extraordinary first sentence of Le protocole compassionnel contains the following passage:

> the body of an old man took possession of my thirty-five-year-old man's frame, it was now likely that because of my loss of strength I had grown much older than my father who has just turned seventy, I'm ninety-five now, like my great-aunt Suzanne who is bed-ridden. (2; translation modified)

> [un corps de vieillard avait pris possession de mon corps d'homme de trente-cinq ans, il était probable que dans la déperdition de mes forces j'avais largement dépassé mon père qui vient d'en avoir soixante-dix, j'ai quatre-vingt-quinze ans comme ma grand-tante Suzanne qui est impotente. (10)]

Such weakness and powerlessness is characteristic of both childhood and old age, and Guibert soon remarks: "I have the feeling I'm a little boy, I have the feeling I am the photo by Eugene Smith of that emaciated old man suffering from radiation sickness . . . I could laugh like some happy, care-free child, the world was upside-down" (PC, 5; translation modified) ["j'avais l'impression d'être un enfant, j'avais l'impression d'être la photo d'Eugene Smith du vieillard irradié et décharné . . . je riais gaiement comme un enfant heureux et insouciant, le monde était renversé" (13)]. If the metaphor of old age seems to correspond more literally to the situation of the narrator, who does not have much longer to live, its juxtaposition with images of childhood places the PWA at both extremities of life, where one is not yet or no longer recognized as a complete human being. Guibert later writes: "In 1990 I am ninety-five, when in fact I was born in 1955. A form of rotation has been set in motion, a gyratory, accelerating movement that has knocked me flat, as if against the revolving wall of a fairground centrifuge, and ground my limbs in a mixer" (94; translation modified) ["En 1990 j'ai quatre-vingt-quinze ans, alors que je suis né en 1955. Une rotation s'est effectuée, un mouvement giratoire qui m'a plaqué comme une centrifugeuse de foire, et a broyé mes membres dans un mixer" (111)]. Decentered and powerless, the diseased subject can no longer claim the hegemonic position of the healthy subject.

Ultimately, looking at himself in the mirror gives the narrator the opportunity to face his own fragmentation every day, his own otherness:

> This confrontation every morning with my nudity in the mirror was a primal experience, lived through again every day, I can't say the prospect helped me to extricate myself from my bed. Nor can I claim I've felt pity for the fellow in the mirror, but it depends, some days I get the feeling he'll make it, because people did come back from Auschwitz, at other times it is obvious he is condemned. (*PC, 7*)

> [Cette confrontation tous les matins avec ma nudité dans la glace était une expérience fondamentale, chaque jour renouvelée, je ne peux pas dire que sa perspective m'aidait à m'extraire de mon lit. Je ne peux pas dire non plus que j'avais de la pitié pour ce type, ça dépend des jours, parfois j'ai l'impression qu'il va s'en sortir puisque des gens sont bien revenus d'Auschwitz, d'autres fois il est clair qu'il est condamné. (15)]

As dramatized by the switch from the first person to the third, the reflection in the mirror figures the otherness in and of the self, the old man, the child, the Holocaust survivor—that body so foreign to the self yet also the self. The recognition of that constitutive otherness, more than anything else, confirms the fracture of the diseased subject. And to the diseased subject corresponds naturally a diseased discourse.

The Discourse of Disease and the Disease of Discourse

In his AIDS novels, Guibert does away with linearity, thus repudiating the idea of a teleological narrative which has framed dominant AIDS discourses. As we discussed earlier, dominant AIDS discourses, whether medical, journalistic, or popular, are always normative. They rest on a certain number of preexisting narrative models—such as the medicalization of homosexuality, degeneracy, or vampire stories—designed to make sense of the epidemic by forcibly inscribing people with HIV or AIDS within the constraints of a teleology. In Guibert's work, however, the chronology of the events that make up the novels is very difficult to reconstruct, as the narrator manages to lose his readers in an inextricable web of anecdotes, dates, memories, and so forth. Furthermore, in *A l'ami*, each "chapter" consists of a paragraph, sometimes even of one single sentence stretching over several pages and randomly mixing several time periods and tenses until the end of the sentence/chapter becomes impossible to predict. In other words, the unstable structure of the novel, reflected on a smaller scale within the sentences, mirrors what Guibert calls "this borderline of uncertainty, so familiar to all sick people everywhere" (*A l'ami*, 3) ["cette frange d'incertitude, qui est commune à tous les malades du monde" (11)]. Such uncertainty, of course, went against the accepted belief at the time that AIDS was invariably fatal.

More powerfully perhaps, the very last "sentence" of *Le protocole compassionnel* directly contradicts the teleology of mainstream AIDS narratives. Guibert writes: "My first film" (199) ["Mon premier film" (227)], where the reader would expect "my last novel." The closing chapter/paragraph of *A l'ami* expresses simultaneously the darkest of despairs and a kind of hope, as the narrator's disappearing body doesn't seem to propel him forward, toward death, but rather back to his childhood to fulfill the long, nostalgic quest that has occupied him for years: "My book is closing in on me. I'm in deep shit. Just how deep do you want me to sink? Hang yourself, Bill! My muscles have melted away. At last my arms and legs are once again as slender as they were when I was a child" (246; translation modified) ["La mise en abîme de mon livre se referme sur moi. Je suis dans la merde. Jusqu'où souhaites-tu me voir sombrer? Pends-toi, Bill! Mes muscles ont fondu. J'ai enfin retrouvé mes jambes et mes bras d'enfant" (267)]. As for the opening sentence of *A l'ami*, "I had AIDS for three months" (1) ["J'ai eu le sida pendant trois mois" (9)], it seems rather incoherent at first because what it denotes is impossible. For Apter, this sentence represents "a certain defiance of the terminal logic imposed on AIDS" (84), which is an accurate reading of it, but soon after she concludes: "The life posture of *dénégation* . . . with its traumatic epistemology of cynicism and suspension of disbelief, shows itself . . . in Guibert's tricks with rhetorical and narratological temporality" (85). But is it really denial?

A l'ami is composed of one hundred chapters, breaking the novel into as many irreconcilable fragments. Dominant AIDS narratives give the illusion of totality, or completion. They have a beginning, a middle, and an end. They provide a structure in which everything can be and eventually will be accounted for. Fragments, on the other hand, acknowledge that something has been so badly broken that it can never be put back together again. One will never be able to "see the whole picture," as the phrase goes, at least not a faithful rendition of it. As hinted by Guibert's entire work, "wholeness" becomes forever pushed back to function only as an originary myth. Finally, fragmentation begs the unanswerable question, What is between the fragments? The unspeakable part of Guibert's "writing of disaster" is, it seems to me, quite different from denial.[21] What Guibert is questioning in his rhetorical choices goes beyond the alleged lethal coherence of AIDS, to destabilize the lethal coherence of discourse itself.

Along with the repositioning of the diseased subject, a new type of discourse on disease can be elaborated. Such discourse, which I propose to call diseased discourse, would not seek to cover the entire field of human experience to extract reified meanings and knowledges. Instead it would acknowledge blanks and silences to figure the constitutive fracture of its subject. It is in that sense that one should understand Guibert's "project of self-revelation and the statement of the unspeakable" (A l'ami, 228; translation modified) ["projet du dévoilement de soi et de l'énoncé de l'indicible" (247)]. For example, after the disastrous fiberoptic exam mentioned earlier, Guibert writes:

> When I got home, I opened my journal and wrote: "Fibroscopy." Nothing else, nothing more, no explanation, no description of the examination and no commentary on my sufferings, it was impossible to put two words together, I was speechless, mouth agape. I had become incapable of recounting my experience. (PC, 48)

> [Chez moi j'ouvris mon journal, et j'y écrivis: "Fibroscopie." Rien d'autre, rien de plus, aucune explication, aucune description de l'examen et aucun commentaire sur ma souffrance, impossible d'aligner deux mots, le sifflet coupé, bouche bée. J'étais devenu incapable de raconter mon expérience. (60)]

Extreme suffering entails the failure of any "explanation," "description," or "commentary." Language, in other words, cannot fulfill its traditional role in the construction of knowledge. Even "aligner deux mots"—literally: put two words side by side in a line—becomes unfeasible. Something in that experience is just impossible to articulate. Yet the scene is there in the book, and the author does exactly what the narrator said could not be done. The unspeakable, then, must be elsewhere.

The scene of the fiberoptic exam constitutes a turning point in the text, folding it in a before-and-after structure. It is after this scene of unparalleled violence that the camcorder begins to appear in the novel, and this camcorder, as we have seen, was the instrument that allowed the construction of a new type of subject. The fiberoptic exam, whose memory runs through everything else after that, becomes the violent fracture, the symbolic point of origin of the diseased subject in the text. In this sense, it stands for that other originary event—the revelation of HIV-positivity. It is in fact that first fracture that has allowed Guibert to radicalize his work, as he says. It is the inaugural moment that shall remain unspoken, in the space between Guibert's illness and its literary account.

In "Plato's Pharmacy," Derrida writes: "Metaphoricity is the logic of contamination and the contamination of logic."[22] And the Latin verb *contaminare* means "to bring into contact with." Contamination, then, is truly the principle governing metaphors, a trope in which the mental image of a thing is brought into contact with the name of another—and vice versa. All discourse originates in this very contamination, including Guibert's novels but also medical discourse. While the latter is entirely occupied with hiding an origin that would delegitimate it, Guibert, on the other hand, explicitly states that without contamination—his own as well as that of his texts—his novels would not exist. The presence of HIV in Guibert's blood is paralleled by the contaminating influence of Austrian writer Thomas Bernhard over his style:

> There's a demon stowed away in my baggage compartment: TB. I've stopped reading these pages to keep the poison from spreading. It's said that each reintroduction of the AIDS virus through bodily fluids—blood, sperm, tears—renews the attack on the already infected patient; perhaps they're just saying that in an effort to contain the damage. (*A l'ami*, 4)

> [Un diable s'est glissé dans mes soutes: T. B. Je me suis arrêté de le lire pour stopper l'empoisonnement. On dit que chaque réinjection du virus du sida par fluides, le sang, le sperme ou les larmes, réattaque le malade déjà contaminé, on prétend peut-être ça pour limiter les dégâts. (12)]

Reading becomes a high-risk behavior that can threaten the plenitude of both the supposedly healthy subject and its discourses. Toward the end of the novel, Guibert writes:

> this Bernhardian metastasis has spread just like the HIV virus at Top Speed . . . through the viral tissues and reflexes of my writing . . . destroying all its personality and natural qualities. . . . I impatiently await the literary vaccine that will deliver me from the spell I purposefully cast

upon myself through Thomas Bernhard, transforming the observation and admiration of his writing . . . into a parodic motif of writing, and into a pathogenic threat, into AIDS. (*A l'ami*, 198–99; translation modified)

[parallèlement donc au virus HIV la métastase bernhardienne s'est propagée à la vitesse grand V dans mes tissus et mes réflexes vitaux d'écriture, elle . . . en détruit tout naturel et toute personnalité . . . j'attends avec impatience le vaccin littéraire qui me délivrera du sortilège que je me suis infligé à dessein par l'entremise de Thomas Bernhard, transformant l'observation et l'admiration de son écriture . . . en motif parodique d'écriture, et en menace pathogène, en sida. (216–17)]

The notions of personality and naturalness Guibert pretends to miss are characteristic of the dominant bourgeois discourse of modernity—from which medical discourse proceeds. But unlike bourgeois writers, Guibert acknowledges the necessity of contamination, as he notes in *Le protocole compassionnel*: "It was apparent that I could not write without admiring someone else's writing" (15) ["Il était clair que je ne pouvais pas écrire sans admirer une écriture" (23)]. In this sense, the HIV/Thomas Bernhard metaphor helps define Guibert's language—and indeed all language—as diseased and infectious. By equating reading and fucking, Guibert reminds his readers that we too may be engaging in risky behavior. Just as Guibert contaminated himself by reading Bernhard, the reader may in turn become contaminated by reading Guibert. As we observed earlier, in *Le protocole compassionnel* the narrator directly addresses the readers in terms of their contamination, asking them if they're enjoying it. Guibert eventually reclaims contamination not only as a destructive but as a productive process. Just like HIV infection, diseased discourse can then spread like an epidemic—which brings me to the subject of gossip.

Gossip, Rumors, and the Margins of Modernity

When *A l'ami* was published, it was warmly received by most critics. Many of these critics, however, saw one major flaw with what they insisted was a *roman à clé*: it contained a lot of gossip, or what writer Michel Braudeau, who reviewed the book in *Le monde*, called "a considerable number of indiscretions" ["un lot considérable d'indiscrétions"].[23] Of course, Muzil, the philosopher who dies of AIDS, who used to hang out in San Francisco's bathhouses and leather bars, who leaves behind a suitcase full of whips and chains, is Michel Foucault, whose open secrets Guibert supposedly revealed for the first time to the public. Of course, Marine, the young movie star falsely rumored to have AIDS, is Isabelle Adjani—to name only the most recognizable ones. According to Braudeau, "certain gossip would be better left to Roger Peyrefitte, who is already peddling it" ["il y a des propos qu'il vaut mieux laisser à Roger Peyrefitte, qui a déjà tout un fond de commerce de la chose"]. The disparaging comparison with author Roger Peyrefitte, a flamboyant Parisian queen, suggests that Braudeau's condemnation of gossip is far from innocent. It defines gossip as an activity of fags unfit for a serious writer.

What Braudeau and others seem to overlook, however, is that the critics who attacked Guibert for gossiping about Foucault seldom failed to reveal the real identities behind the pseudonyms, or to mention the unwholesome yet juicy bits, thus engaging themselves in a practice they claimed to condemn. Moreover, as the content of these reviews demonstrates, it was largely because of its gossip that *A l'ami* got so much public exposure in the first place. It is also obvious that literary and academic circles in Paris and elsewhere had long gossiped about Foucault's tastes in sex and the cause of his death. Again, both were open secrets. And to be quite specific, Didier Eribon was the first to mention all this in print in his biography of Foucault, published a year before Guibert's fictional account.[24] Would it be fair to say, then, that some critics and academics were so angry because, thanks to Guibert's success and TV appearances, gossip about Foucault started to spread outside the small authorized circles of experts and into the larger popular culture? In this case, their attacks would not be so much a condemnation of gossip per se (which, coming from literary and intellectual circles would be the epitome of hypocrisy), but rather a dispute over something like class privileges maintained by secrecy.

Ross Chambers has observed that secrecy is indeed connected to the idea of power: "The sharing of secrets defines social groups by the simple criterion of inclusion and exclusion: there are those who are 'in on' the secret and those who aren't, or to complexify, those who know the secret, those who know there is a secret but are not permitted to share it, and those who are ignorant both of the existence of a secret and its content. In this way, secrecy has obvious links with the distribution of power."[25] By going public, that is, by sharing the secret with everyone who cares to read, Guibert broke what Chambers calls "the rule limiting . . . repeatability to appropriate hearers" ("Histoire d'Oeuf," 69). He upset the distribution of power and threatened the boundaries and privileges of the community previously (per)formed by the gossip—or sharing of the secret—about Foucault. To limit the damage, they could only pretend that Foucault's sex life and the cause of his death were in fact irrelevant information and that Guibert had accomplished nothing.

But Guibert's gesture allows for a democratized appropriation of Foucault by a new community. In that community, the circumstances of his death could actually be very relevant to someone who might not even have read Foucault, someone for whom Foucault is less a major philosopher than a famous gay man who died of AIDS. It is precisely because Foucault's homosexuality was dismissed as trivial that circulating such information was defined (and condemned) as gossip. Two factors, therefore, explain the reaction of so many of Guibert's critics: a fear of losing the power granted to them by the sharing of the secret; and homophobia.

In Guibert's text, gossip provides queer readers with a familiar mode of communication: gossip has been for many of us an inevitable and even vital activity. According to Douglas Crimp, "The most fundamental need gossip has served for queers is that of the construction—and reconstruction—of our identities."[26] Indeed, gossip allows the circulation of certain types of information and knowledge that, until the development of a commercial gay press, had been almost entirely excluded from the media. To the extent that gossip contributes to the construction of queer subjectivities, rejecting it amounts to shoving homosexuality back into the strict confines of the private sphere. Patricia Meyer Spacks stresses that gossip can indeed subvert the dichotomy between public and private spheres. She writes: "Often articulated in intimate association, gossip yet speaks for groups: sometimes small sub-societies, sometimes larger communities. It circulates and ponders facts of private existence. Blurring the boundaries between the personal and the widely known, it implicitly challenges the separation of realms . . . assumed in modern times."[27] The consequences of this blurring of boundaries are crucial in the context of AIDS, which has forever modified the way queer identities are constructed.

From the outset AIDS has provided a fertile terrain for gossip and rumors. It was first associated with (homo)sexuality and drugs, scandalous behaviors that were already the subject matter of gossip. But more important, gossip and rumors began to circulate through the silences and half-truths of official stories. For example, when one reads in the newspaper obituaries that so-and-so, hairdresser to the stars, died of complications from pneumonia, gossip fills in the blanks. It keeps official stories from being reified as normative knowledge, be it scientific, historical, or biographical.

A good example of this is the rumor about French entertainer Thierry Le Luron, an episode that contributed a great deal to public perceptions of AIDS in France. The time was the mid-1980s, when knowledge about AIDS was still very uncertain, and no French celebrity had yet gone public about being HIV-positive: in other words, the context was ideal for rumors. A few weeks after Rock Hudson's death in 1985, Thierry Le Luron, a young and somewhat openly gay Parisian entertainer, was rumored to have AIDS after he abruptly canceled a series of performances, was hospitalized, and made unexplained trips to the United States.[28] Le Luron publicly denied being sick, and blamed Parisian gay circles for spreading the rumor.[29] In October 1986, Léon Schwartzenberg, a famous cancer specialist and one-time government official with a reputation for "telling it like it is," announced that his famous patient had cancer, not AIDS. On 13 November, Le Luron died.

What is striking in this episode is that, by and large, the public didn't believe the word of the famous doctor, and today it is accepted as common knowledge that Le Luron died of AIDS. Gossip and rumors have effectively undermined the authority of official/medical discourse by maintaining a competing version of the facts, a version that has ultimately prevailed. In this case, gossip and rumors have allowed the crucial elaboration of AIDS knowledge, and have transformed the overall cultural construction of the epidemic in France. Indeed, as science journalist Jérôme Strazzula rightly observes, Le Luron's death marked a turning point, after which French celebrities who had HIV or AIDS began to go public about it.[30]

But exactly what kind of knowledge does gossip construct? Guibert's fictional account of the Adjani rumor shows how it mirrored dominant AIDS narratives. First, the rumor of Marine's AIDS seemed to give full meaning to past events in retrospect, thus echoing a widespread tendency in early AIDS discourses. Second, it "confirmed" nearly all the accepted clichés about AIDS transmission:

> One day the hot tip is that she caught it shooting up with her brother, who's a little junkie, the next day someone else swears she got it from a blood transfusion, and a third opinion gave it to her through her no-good Yank, who's a first class bisexual party animal, and so on. (*A l'ami,* 116; translation modified)

> [Un jour un informateur colporte qu'elle l'a attrapé en se piquant avec son frère, qui est un petit junkie, le lendemain une autre source d'information assure qu'elle a été contaminée lors d'une transfusion de sang, un troisième écho le lui refilera par son amerloque à la noix, qui est un partouzeur bisexuel de première, et cetera. (130)]

With its mentions of drugs, blood transfusion, homosexuality, and the United States, the passage is a striking summary of early AIDS construction in France.

This suggests that the rumor is not an aberrant outgrowth on "rational" AIDS discourse but a rather faithful repetition of it, albeit in a parodic and destabilizing mode. Finally, when Guibert writes "un troisième écho le lui refilera," the use of the active voice suggests that language not only constructs the image of the PWA but also spreads it. As Guibert's syntactical choice emphasizes, Marine is contaminated by the rumor itself. Ultimately, the actual rumors about Adjani and Le Luron were cofactors, as it were, of the onset of AIDS in the French collective consciousness.

When I wrote earlier that gossip fills in the blanks, I did not mean that it necessarily fills them with the truth. If we agree that, regardless of the facts, what we call "the true story" is simply the narrative that prevails in the end, gossip keeps reminding us that no narrative can ever fully prevail. We the public do not know for certain that Le Luron died of AIDS. We cannot be sure either that Guibert told us the truth about Foucault. In fact, the way gossip spreads has become a classic joke. As the information circulates, participants tend to add details to the original story or fact so that it soon bears no resemblance to what it first was. Gossip is a transformation of narrative and a narrative of transformation. It is made to look like the inverted mirror image of the traditional process of normal scientific progress in which facts and discoveries are piled up in order to get closer and closer to the complete knowledge of the truth. What it really tells us, though, is that the knowledge of gossip is not normalizing. It is unstable, uncertain, and temporary, and as such, not unlike most knowledge about AIDS, an epidemic still ruled by doubts and questions, such as: How safe is safe sex? Can I believe him when he says he's HIV-negative? Are we sometimes tested without our knowledge? How did it all really start? Will we ever find a cure? Are treatments making PWAs sicker? How long will combination-therapies work? Living in a world with AIDS means managing uncertainty one way or another. Gossip and rumors are ways we do just that, and, because their mode of dissemination is structurally epidemic, they are particularly helpful to the communities most concerned about the epidemic in the first place.

On a less global level, gossip and rumors simultaneously disseminate information and structure communities. In a word, they relate, in both senses of the term: they tell a story, and by doing so establish a relationship. Practically, gossip and rumors construct alternative networks of communication for those who do not have a direct role in shaping official discourse and policy. In *Epistemology of the Closet,* Eve Kosofsky Sedgwick rightly points out that gossip has been "immemorially associated in European thought with servants, with effeminate and gay men, with all women" (23); and the list could go on to include other categories of people, such as prison inmates, whose common characteristic is to be excluded from the elaboration of official discourse and/or defined as out-siders. Rumors also tend to spread easily in outlawed communities, such as those of undocumented immigrants or drug users. As it turns out, this list re-sembles closely that of the communities most affected by AIDS in Western countries.

Writing about a video produced by lesbians and centered around the absent character of country singer Dolly Parton, long rumored to be gay, Crimp con-cludes: "Dolly Parton may be the subject of the gossip, but the subjectivity rep-resented in the video is that of the lesbians who gossip among themselves about Dolly. What matters is *their* visibility" ("Right On, Girlfriend!" 12; original em-phasis). In *A l'ami* the character of Muzil plays the same role. What matters in the story of Muzil's AIDS is not so much what it says about the character as what it says about the narrator and, eventually, the readers. Referring to his diary en-tries about Muzil, but probably anticipating the criticism he would face for his book, Guibert writes:

> What right did I have to record all that? What right did I have to use friendship in such a mean fashion? And with someone I adored with all my heart? And then I sensed—it's extraordinary—a kind of vision, or vertigo, that gave me complete authority, putting me in charge of these ignoble transcripts and legitimizing them by revealing to me . . . that I was completely entitled to do this since it wasn't so much my friend's last agony I was describing as it was my own, which was waiting for me and would be just like his. (*A l'ami,* 91)

> [De quel droit écrivais-je tout cela? De quel droit faisais-je de telles en-tailles à l'amitié? Et vis-à-vis de quelqu'un que j'adorais de tout mon coeur? Je ressentis alors, c'était inouï, une sorte de vision, ou de vertige, qui m'en donnait les pleins pouvoirs, qui me délégaient à ces transcrip-tions ignobles et qui les légitimaient en m'annonçant . . . que j'y étais pleinement habilité car ce n'était pas tant l'agonie de mon ami que j'étais en train de décrire que l'agonie qui m'attendait, et qui serait identique. (101–2)]

Critics often make the mistake of reading this passage at face value. In fact, as is often the case in this narrative structure of dual autobiography so characteristic of AIDS testimonials, the depiction of the friend's illness and death also provides the narrator with a counterexample. In this case, unlike Muzil, Guibert will not let himself be victimized by doctors and relatives. Muzil/Foucault, then, allows the narrator/author to try to make sense of his own experience, and the readers to try to make sense of their own. In the process, a community is formed. The same could be said of the rumor about Marine/Adjani. It is of course a good and important thing that Isabelle Adjani did not get sick and die, so that she could go on to make *Diabolique;* but in a cultural sense, it doesn't matter so much that the rumor was actually false, and that Marine/Adjani didn't really have AIDS after all. What matters is that the rumor did help to shape our understanding of the AIDS crisis. Hence the importance of Guibert's indiscretions and his use of easily recognizable celebrities as fictional characters.

In "Gossip and the Novel," Ross Chambers writes: "Fictive productions serve, like gossip, to identify and explore our values through the production of special, noteworthy, extraordinary or scandalous ('tellable') cases: as such, they are an important mode of sociological and psychological theorizing. But when it masquerades as the true, the fictive . . . can become a form of symbolic, sometimes actual victimization. Members of minoritized social groups (blacks, women, gays . . .) daily fall victim to what is, in effect, the prevailing gossip about them" (215). Guibert's intelligence and talent is precisely to appropriate a form of narrative construction of knowledge (actually two forms that are closely related, as Chambers points out: gossip and the novel) that had been used to perform exclusion, and, as drag does with gender, redirect it against the dominant system of representation. While there is no denying that gossip and rumors can be extremely malicious and harmful, scandal, for Guibert, is elsewhere.

For Guibert, the unacceptable scandal is not in his gossipy novels but in the dominant representations of people with AIDS. In *Le protocole compassionnel,* the narrator is wondering what he could videotape for the film he is preparing. During one of his many hospital stays, as he is surrounded by fellow patients, he concludes: "I told myself that one could never film these walking corpses as I had once thought of doing after the television producer's proposal, that it would be a real scandal, an uninteresting scandal" (*PC,* 36; translation modified) ["Je me suis dit qu'on ne pourrait pas filmer ces cadavres ambulants comme j'y avais pensé un moment à cause de la proposition de la productrice de télé, que ce serait finalement un vrai scandale, un scandale inintéressant" (46)]. One is reminded here of the way PWAs were typically portrayed by the media in the 1980s so as to create an unbridgeable split between them and the viewers.[31] On the other hand, gossip, the interesting scandal, constructs a community of listeners, or readers in this case. The hostility of the reviews in *Le monde* and elsewhere may be explained by the fact that Guibert's texts tend to suppress the safe distance that the theoretically (that is, until stated otherwise) healthy, heterosexual critic intends to maintain between himself and the narrator with AIDS. Guibert invites his readers to gossip and to partake in an activity traditionally associated with women and men who look—and talk—like them. To dismiss gossip altogether means to refuse not only to participate in the communal ritual of the excluded, but also, and mainly, to refuse to acknowledge that it is a community in the first place, and one which uses gossip as a tool for empowerment. In the specific context of the AIDS crisis and Guibert's novels, dismissing gossip and condemning rumors are ways of protecting oneself from contamination— from both HIV and queerness. Instead of consenting to unsafe reading and letting himself be infected by Guibert's text, the critic from *Le monde* prefers to read with a condom.

Finally, I would like to return to the subject of "the subject," and specifically to its relation with gossip. And to do so, I find it valuable to refer back to Michel Foucault—not to the gay man who died of AIDS in Paris on 25 June 1984 at the age of 58, not to the fictional re-creation of this man in Hervé Guibert's novels under the name Muzil, but to Michel Foucault's writings. In his essay "What Is an Author?" Foucault writes: "How can one reduce the great peril, the great danger with which fiction threatens our world? The answer is: One can reduce it with the author. The author allows a limitation of *the cancerous and dangerous proliferation of significations* within a world where one is thrifty not only with one's resources and riches, but also with one's discourses and their significations. The author is the principle of thrift in the proliferation of meaning" (158–59; my emphasis). According to Foucault, "The coming into being of the notion of 'author' constitutes the privileged moment of *individualization* in the history of ideas, knowledge, literature, philosophy, and the sciences" (141; original emphasis). To follow up on Foucault's cancer metaphor, one could add that the (literary) author as individual heroic subject is endowed with the same, albeit metaphoric, functions as the modern doctor: to stop the spread of a disease potentially damaging to society as a whole. (As we discussed earlier in this book, Zola took this metaphor quite seriously.) But what about authorship outside the field of literature? Foucault points out that in the Middle Ages literary texts did not need an individual author to be accepted as literature, while scientific texts had to be attributed to an author to be considered valid. Finally, after the seventeenth or eighteenth century, the situations were reversed: "Scientific discourses began to be received for themselves, in the anonymity of an established and always redemonstrable truth" (149).

One could wonder, however, to what degree the anonymity of scientific truth is still operating in the age of AIDS. Uncertainty about HIV and AIDS, still so prevalent in the public mind, and the absence of a radical cure or vaccine almost two decades after the crisis began, have shaken the blind trust Western societies had placed in medicine since the nineteenth century. Even before AIDS, numerous critics, including Foucault, of course, had begun to expose medical discourses as ideological constructs, as narratives. These critiques were radicalized in the current context, and they destabilized the hegemony of medical discourse by making it one of the many competing narratives with which we try to make sense of what is happening to us. This does not mean, obviously, that the content of medical discourse is now universally seen as fictional. What has become increasingly accepted, however, is the idea that medical discourses are elaborated in ways that are not unlike fiction, that they may even be informed by fiction, and that science and literature may not be as neatly separated as previously thought. Hence the return of the authors. Luc Montagnier, Robert Gallo, Willy Rozenbaum, Jacques Leibowitch, Anthony Fauci, and David Ho are not only authors of books, they are also signature names that are repeatedly summoned to authenticate "AIDS truths." There seldom is an AIDS-related show on French TV without Montagnier, and Fauci and Ho have become fixtures on American television news shows. These individual names signify authority in all senses of the term.

Now consider gossip and rumors about AIDS. They are constantly dismissed as dangerous fictions in a domain where "knowing the facts" is supposed to save our lives. (But, as Chambers points out, it is when fiction masquerades as truth that there is danger.) Interestingly, what characterizes these fictions is that nobody knows for sure where they came from. In other words, they cannot be attributed to a single author. If they were, they would cease to be gossip or rumors and become libel. "[T]he cancerous and dangerous proliferation of significations" has been, one hopes, effectively ended by the attribution of the fiction to an author. Hence the urge to find a single culprit to blame, such as Guibert, for example. But what is particularly striking in the case of A l'ami is the critics' insistence on Foucault instead of the fictional Muzil, that is, on reading Guibert's text as nonfiction. And as we have seen, this truth factor was used precisely to deny Guibert's novel the qualities of true literature. As one critic wrote:

> He tells and reveals what his friends wanted to keep silent about themselves, and he decides that the headlines of *France-Dimanche* are worth more than the litotes and equivocations for which our language has been celebrated, and that allow us to say everything without naming anything.

> [Il raconte et révèle ce que ses amis voulaient taire sur eux-mêmes et décide que les en-têtes de France-Dimanche valent mieux que la litote ou ces phrases équivoques qui firent la gloire de notre langue et qui permettent de tout dire sans nommer.][32]

And again, the depiction of Guibert as author of gossip is parallel to the dis-

Conclusion

French Universalism and the
Question of Community

During a demonstration organized by ACT UP-New York, film historian Vito Russo concluded his speech with these words: "After we kick the shit out of this disease, I intend to be alive to kick the shit out of this system so that it will never happen again."[1] In the French context, Mathieu Duplay, a former spokesperson for ACT UP-Paris, once defined the association's new brand of activism as follows:

> We are not fighting for a new model of democracy. Of course we do demand that certain systems be reformed, such as the prison and education systems, for example. But we are concerned, first and foremost, with the immediate problem: AIDS. As for reforms, we'll see about that in due course!

> [Nous ne luttons pas pour un nouveau modèle de démocratie. Bien sûr que nous réclamons une réforme des systèmes, carcéral ou éducatif notamment. Mais nous nous occupons avant tout du problème immédiat: le sida. Pour les réformes, nous verrons après!][2]

But to what extent can the fight against AIDS be chronologically separated from the fight for a different type of society, as both Russo and Duplay seem to suggest? When the latter states that "ACT UP provides a structure to rethink a citizen's global position from his/her HIV-positivity" ["ACT UP est avant tout une structure qui permet de repenser la position globale du citoyen à partir de sa séropositivité" (56)], doesn't that automatically entail a rethinking of how citizenship is defined for all? And doesn't that, therefore, imply a rethinking of what defines the nation as a whole? In fact, by bringing the question of communities to the forefront of the current debates on French identity, the AIDS crisis and its responses may already have contributed to triggering a radical change in France's definitions of citizenship and nationhood.

In April 1996, a controversy erupted around the displays of rainbow flags in the Marais, the old Parisian neighborhood home to what may or may not be the gay community. Indeed, what was soon to be known as the *affaire des drapeaux,* the flag controversy, signaled a new chapter in the debate over the existence and status of minority communities in French society. A neighborhood association circulated a petition opposing the mass display of the international gay emblem by businesses. Pierre-Charles Krieg, the mayor of the fourth *arrondissement* at the time, forwarded the complaint to the police, who began a systematic campaign of harassment against gay bars, with the unavowed purpose of shutting down as many as possible in order to prevent the Marais from becoming a predominantly gay neighborhood. Eventually a compromise was reached between the city of Paris and gay business owners: rainbow flags were allowed to hang only during Gay Pride celebrations.[3] A year later the Ordre des pharmaciens, the national association of pharmacists, banned the gay-owned pharmacy in the Marais from displaying the rainbow flag or any other identifiable symbol of gayness, and allowed only a supposedly more universal flag bearing the red ribbon of AIDS solidarity. Why did these incidents trigger such controversy? As we shall see, competing AIDS discourses are at the heart of the question of community in France today. To conclude this book, then, I would like to show how the AIDS epidemic in France is inextricably linked to the tensions between opposing conceptions of the place of communities in the Republic. I will briefly consider the television fund-raising show *Sidaction* to illustrate how any long-term solution to the AIDS crisis can only entail a radical alteration of the republican model of universal integration.

Although the incidents I described barely made national headlines, they are central to understanding the identity crisis that has been haunting the French republic of late. To be sure, this crisis is not entirely new. In fact, the *affaire des drapeaux* reminds us of another *affaire du drapeau* when, during the unstable period preceding the Third Republic, the count of Chambord, heir to the throne, could have seized power. But he stubbornly refused to give up the royal white flag for the tricolor, thus ruining the last chance for the restoration of the monarchy, and inaugurating the longest republic France has ever known. The official ban on what were perceived as ostentatious signs of collective identity also directly echoes the much more recent (1989) *affaire des foulards*, or veil controversy, when several Muslim girls were not allowed to attend classes in public schools as long as they refused to remove their veils. The incident ignited a heated national debate on the issues of cultural pluralism and national identity. A striking aspect of this debate was that it did not reproduce the traditional Left-Right polarization so typical of French political culture. Instead it revealed a split among those on the Left, as exemplified by the "first couple." While François Mitterrand defended a strict republican stance on secular schools, his wife Danielle expressed a more multiculturalist viewpoint. At stake was more than a presidential marriage, but the definition of the French Left for the future. Finally, in 1994, the government banned all *signes ostentatoires* of religion in public schools. Nearly a decade later, it is the gay community's turn to find itself at the heart of what I think is essentially the same controversy.

While immigration and homosexuality resonate differently from each other in French culture, the debates around them have recently taken similar directions. In a now infamous speech, Jacques Chirac, then mayor of Paris, talked about the "smells" of foreigners disturbing French neighbors. He later explained that he was referring to the smells of foreign cuisine. But since in French public discourse "cuisine" often means "culture," we understand that it is foreign culture that is a factor of social disharmony. Today, straight neighbors in the Marais complain about boys who, while sitting on public benches, give the expression "French kissing" a slightly different meaning. Interestingly enough, the article in *Le monde* recounting this particular "incident" is titled "The gay flag hangs over the rue Sainte-Croix-de-la-Bretonnerie" ["Le drapeau gay flotte rue Sainte-Croix-de-la-Bretonnerie"], a metaphor of foreign invasion. The same week, *L'événement du jeudi* described the Marais as the "headquarters of the homosexual lobby" ["quartier général du lobby homosexuel"], mixing a military trope with an allusion to American-style politics. Not unlike Arab and Muslim cultures, the emerging gay "culture" is described as essentially un-French and unassimilable. Only when confined to the strict boundaries of the private sphere is homosexuality deemed acceptable by the Republic.

This traditional view of the republican model of nationhood defines French citizenship as a contract resulting from a political will, from the convergence of free, individual decisions to live together according to a core of basic universal principles.[4] As Ernest Renan wrote in "Qu'est-ce qu'une nation?" ["What Is a Nation?"] a nation is constituted by "the consent, the clearly expressed desire to keep on living together" ["le consentement, le désir clairement exprimé de continuer la vie ensemble" (307)] or what he calls "a daily plebiscite" ["un plébiscite de tous les jours" (307)]. Conversely, "race, language, interests, religious affinity, geography, military necessities" ["la race, la langue, les intérêts, l'affinité religieuse, la géographie, les nécessités militaires" (305)], by themselves, are not valid principles on which to build a nation. Consequently, the model of the "République une et indivisible" does not recognize communities as political actors within the Republic: there must be nothing between the state and the individual. Specific cultures and religious practices are protected as long as they do not conflict with core principles and are circumscribed to the private sphere. Indeed, this is the only way individual freedom can be guaranteed.

While this framework was intended to deal mostly with the questions of foreign immigration and religion, it has recently been extended to include sexual orientation. Since the early 1980s, homosexuality has been depenalized, and the so-called general public is said to be increasingly accepting of it. The tragedy of AIDS and the visible mobilization of gays and lesbians have undoubtedly played a part in this newly gained sympathy; a sympathy, however, that is subject to the same rules of appropriate republican behavior as foreignness or religion: if it is to be tolerated within the Republic, gayness—or rather, homosexuality—must not form the basis of a collective identity or a sort of intermediate political entity.

But in our postindustrial societies this unitarian model is going through a period of profound crisis. According to Alain Touraine, the world is pulled in opposite directions.[5] Globalization—in French, *mondialisation*—has made the economy less and less dependent on the nation-state, creating deep national anxieties. In reaction to this radical loss of identity, a reactive force has begun to privilege a return to communities based on cultural homogeneity. Religious fundamentalisms, ethnic cleansing in the former Yugoslavia, and the rise of the extreme Right in Europe are recent manifestations of such cultural relativism, or *communautarisme*.

The debate around the place of communities in French society can be understood in these terms. The veil controversy dramatized the tension between what were seen as two incompatible responses to the national anxiety: integration or separatism. More recently, the controversy over the legitimacy of the gay community in France has been polarized along the same lines: "Communautarisme ou républicanisme?" asks the monthly gay magazine *Ex aequo*. For its opponents, the notion of a gay community threatens the boundary between public and private spheres, a boundary on which individual freedom rests. The

(hypothetical) gay community is perceived as a factor of increased social fragmentation because it relies on difference rather than on a unifying political will.[6]

This is the thesis of Frédéric Martel's thick and impressive-looking 1996
book *Le rose et le noir*. Although it was widely, and rightly, criticized for being
self-serving, theoretically antiquated, and just plain homophobic, the book enjoyed a tremendous success, and can be credited for triggering the whole debate
about the question of community. It also laid out its terms in a particularly vicious way. There was one aspect of Martel's study that attracted everybody's attention and was used as its main sales pitch: the gay community, he claimed, was
so taken by paranoid delusions of universal homophobia that it turned down
the prompt and generous help of the government and medical establishment
and was therefore largely responsible for the spread of AIDS. These accusations
were then used to justify the book's denunciation of *communautarisme* as both
criminal and suicidal. Adding a semblance of credibility to this thesis was the
fact that Martel is himself gay, thus validating accusations against gays in the
straight press.[7] *Communautarisme*, then, appears so monstrous that it threatens
to destroy not only the Republic but also the subgroup it is designed to protect. Again, the French model of republican integration is presented as the only
salvation.

This strict polarization, however, is untenable. Etienne Balibar, Maxim Silverman, and Michel Wieviorka, to name a few, have shown how the contractual
model of nationhood is always already undermined by its own essentialization,
that is, by the insistence on the Frenchness of the integrationist model, and indeed of republican universalism.[8] The indivisible Republic and its divisive minorities are in fact inextricably bound. As Silverman writes: "The frontiers (both
geographical and metaphorical) defining the nation-state and minorities are
produced at the same time and by the *same* process" (19; original emphasis). In
other words, the Republic invents the very communities it condemns, and essentially in the same terms with which it invented itself.

In fact, the republican model needs to construct a homogeneous other
against which to define itself and hide its internal contradictions. The German
model of citizenship, based on ethnicity, used to play that role, and it is still often presented as the antithesis of the French model.[9] As I have discussed in the
first two chapters of this book, that is certainly the way the republican Left saw
it during the Third Republic, when a vibrant and newly united Germany was
looked upon with a mix of fear, contempt, and envy. Today, it is against the
United States that the French model is measured. The shift has a lot to do with
what France perceives to be the biggest threat to its cultural integrity at a given

historical moment—the *ligne bleue des Vosges* one day, EuroDisney the next. Hence the tendency in France today to have the words *républicanisme* and *communautarisme* followed by *à la française* or *à l'américaine,* respectively. The United States is commonly described as a hopelessly fragmented society, composed of separatist communities at war with each other and imposing their particularisms at the expense of national unity. The fact that, like modern France, the United States was performed into existence by a solemn declaration of free political will seems to be forgotten. And so is the absence of consensus within American society on the issue of multiculturalism. Today, the French national narrative needs to construct the "American model" as radically different, that is, as homogeneous and uncontested. Thanks to the built-in ambiguity of such dichotomies, the intended effect is that the French model will absorb the qualities of its polar opposite so that it too will appear to be homogeneous and uncontested.

The same strategy, and for the same reasons, is also directed inward, and these characteristics are attributed to the various internal communities, often criticized as nations within the nation. Late-nineteenth-century anti-Semitism was an example of such rhetoric. In today's context, the first example that comes to mind is that of North Africans, whether legally French or not. The rhetoric is simple: they are depicted as either full-fledged French citizens—which implies giving up all other cultural allegiances in the public sphere—or as Islamic fundamentalists—an even more potent symbol of un-Frenchness than is the United States.[10] The way the gay community experienced the onset of AIDS in France was framed by the same impossible choice. The initial period of total inaction, referred to as *dédramatisation,* was rationalized by the idea that there is no such thing as a gay identity or a gay community in France; therefore the idea that a virus could strike gay men collectively is absurd. Any claim to the contrary would be irrational, un-French, and could lead to collective hysteria *à l'américaine.*[11]

In Hervé Guibert's *A l'ami qui ne m'a pas sauvé la vie,* Muzil exclaims: "A cancer that would hit only homosexuals, no, that's too good to be true, I could just die laughing!" (13) ["Un cancer qui toucherait exclusivement les homosexuels, non, ce serait trop beau pour être vrai, c'est à mourir de rire" (21)]. Epidemiology, as we know, tells a different story. As I mentioned earlier, if, presumably, everybody *can* get AIDS, not everybody will. It could be argued, then, that by refusing to conceive communities otherwise than in essentialized terms in order to deny their existence within the Republic, France could not understand AIDS, an epidemic inseparable from, although not limited to, the existence of marginalized communities.[12] In other words, France applied its own founding narrative of universal equality to HIV itself, as if the virus were to abide by the "Declaration of the Rights of Man and the Citizen."

Yet one could also argue that there was in fact a concurrent underlying cultural belief in the existence of a distinct gay identity and community, and that the vague hope that the epidemic would remain confined within that undesirable community explains the period of inaction. What may appear to be a contradiction really reflects a tension inherent in the construction of homosexuality in modern French culture, where the homosexual is at the same time an individual citizen with a right to his private sex life, and a distinct and despised species—to use Foucault's terminology.[13] Gay identity, it seems, does and does not exist as a working category in French society.

This gives us an additional argument against Martel's accusations that the gay community is responsible for the spread of AIDS in the 1980s. In fact, it has long been observed that gay activism in France largely disbanded after Mitterrand's first election in 1981, when nearly all demands were met. The year 1981, we recall, is also the year when the first reports on AIDS were published. Soon after that, the community evolved mostly into a highly commercialized Parisian scene. In fact, if Gay Pride parades can be seen as good indicators of the social vitality of the gay community, it is important to notice that, as club owners progressively took control of the yearly marches, attendance plummeted steadily until the early 1990s, when ACT UP-Paris began to reenergize the community. In addition, the few militants still active in the 1980s were, for the most part, former members of the FHAR (Front Homosexuel d'Action Révolutionnaire) or the GLH (Groupe de Libération Homosexuelle). They belonged to a tradition that favored the radical subversion of sexual norms rather than the affirmation of a separate identity in what they called a ghetto.[14] The separatist gay community blamed for the spread of AIDS in the early years simply did not exist. If French gays were late in organizing collective responses to the epidemic, it wasn't, as Martel claims, because of their misplaced allegiance to a separatist community, which they largely rejected, but precisely because they behaved like good, republican Frenchmen.

In the current debate, the gay community is made to embody all the cultural anxieties of the French republic. Not unlike fast-food franchises and imported English words, the rainbow flags are criticized as signs of Americanization, threatening to turn the oldest Parisian neighborhood into the Castro. The flag controversy, then, may be a recent chapter in what many in France see as a cultural showdown against the United States. Logically, "gay culture" is also perceived as a supranational and increasingly uniform lifestyle. It has its symbols, its vacation spots, its use of English as lingua franca, its music, its porn culture, et cetera.[15] In other words, the "gay lifestyle" is emblematic of *mondialisation.* But, as we have seen, it is also exemplary of *communautarisme,* which is the opposite and equally threatening tendency. In short, the "gay community" as it is depicted in the current debate is a rhetorical construction within the republican narrative of Frenchness. It is simultaneously an assertion of identity and a sign of loss of identity, in this case, national identity. It is made to occupy both extremes of the spectrum in order for the republican model to appear, by contrast, as the only reasonable alternative.[16]

On 6 June 1996, these tensions were played out on live television during the second *Sidaction,* which has become a central part of AIDS discourse in France. Held for the first time in 1994, the *Sidaction* is a national fund-raising event, and the first two editions were broadcast simultaneously during prime time by all French television networks. Each show lasted for several hours and was hosted by popular TV personalities. In addition to testimonies from people with AIDS or engaged in the fight against AIDS, it included singers and movie stars appealing to the generosity of viewers. The event itself was preceded by intense media coverage and solicitations for donations almost everywhere. For about a week, the entire country appeared united in its solidarity with people with HIV and AIDS. Every French person, it seemed, was wearing a red ribbon.

The opening segment of the 1996 show set the tone for the evening, with a brief, stylish montage showing a number of people with HIV and AIDS. Through words and images we can figure out that they are a mother and her adult son, children, a straight couple, two brothers, a family, and another straight couple. No social context is provided, and, especially, no kind of collective identification. The message is simple, and has been at the heart of nearly all national prevention campaigns in France: everybody can get AIDS, and the social exclusion of those affected is wrong and un-French. The direct consequence of this message is to construct the disease within the framework of the republican model: AIDS is conceptualized only at the levels of the individual and the nation as a whole, not in terms of intermediate communities. As usual, however, the universal turns out to be the generalization of one particular viewpoint to the exclusion of all others: everybody in the opening segment is white and defined in a heterosexual context.

A bit later, the first person to be interviewed live is a middle-aged, HIV-negative, white woman whose daughter died of AIDS a few years before, and who is now raising three grandchildren, two of whom are HIV-positive. It is in their name that she is appearing on the show. After praising her courage and insisting that there was "no reason" for this grandmother to have to deal with AIDS that way because she had "nothing to do with all that," Jean-Marie Cavada, the interviewer and main presenter of the *Sidaction,* finally calls her "an obvious symbol of the havoc wreaked by this disease" ["un symbole évident des ravages de cette maladie"]. Two conclusions can be drawn from this telling example of the universalizing of AIDS: first, it reinforces the notion of risk groups it was supposed to debunk; and then it constructs atypical cases as "obvious symbols" of AIDS, like a white, HIV-negative grandmother. Once again, the discourse of universal inclusion performs exclusion.

In fact, for the first fifty minutes of the broadcast, the audience gets to listen to all sorts of people, such as families who have lost a loved one to the disease, members of various foundations, doctors, a cabinet minister, and celebrities. With the exception of the opening montage, the only PWAs we see appear on videos of people who participated in the previous *Sidaction* and who have since died. In about an hour, AIDS is thus rewritten as a tale of family tragedy, medical heroism, and government compassion. When the first PWAs are finally introduced live on the set, in a brief segment where each one barely gets the chance to speak, the main topic is the issue of straight couples who want to have children when one of the two is HIV-positive. Those who are presumably gay do not talk about it, and IV drug users are in fact *former* IV drug users presented as admirable for giving up their addiction—which means, for renouncing their membership in a separate (and illegal) community and rejoining the rest of the nation.[17]

As for AIDS in the DOM-TOM (Départements d'Outre-Mer et Territoires d'Outre-Mer), the viewers have to wait until around 11:30 P.M. before being able to see a three-minute story on Martinique, followed by a two-minute live interview with a doctor from French Guiana. From the set-up of the segment on Martinique, we are supposed to understand that the Caribbean island must be representative of all French overseas territories. And, to some extent, it is. In the DOM-TOM, the rates of HIV and AIDS are higher than the national average. French Guiana, for example, has a rate of HIV infection roughly equal to that of Paris. Since the story addresses the causes of the problem, one would expect the reporter to make the obvious connection. What else do these territories, so distant geographically, so different culturally, have in common, beyond their high rate of HIV and AIDS, if not the fact that they are French overseas territories? But instead of analyzing the cause-and-effect relationship between economic disempowerment and the spread of AIDS, the story focuses on cultural taboos supposedly inherent to Caribbean culture. After explaining that AIDS is a serious problem in Martinique, the metropolitan-accented voice-over adds: "But nobody talks about it. In a society where everybody knows everybody, the disease is taboo, even though one advocates solidarity as an essential value of Caribbean society to overcome adversity" ["Mais on n'en parle pas. Au sein d'une société où tout le monde se connaît, la maladie est taboue, même si, par ailleurs, on prône la solidarité comme valeur essentielle de la société antillaise pour surmonter les épreuves"]. And a little later, the following comment on the bigoted initial response of the Catholic church: "Here, the influence of the Church isn't neutral" ["Ici, le poids de l'Église n'est pas neutre"]. Martinique, then, is presented as a self-contained, village-like society, dominated by taboos and excessive religious influence. It is a different "society" with its own "essential values." Despite the fact that the 1946 *départementalisation* was supposed to make Martinique the equal of Tarn-et-Garonne in the eyes of the Republic, it is still simultaneously constructed as a radically essentialized Other. In the context of AIDS, this construction has the effect of exonerating French colonial domination from any responsibility for the seriousness of the epidemic, while blaming the spread of AIDS precisely on the un-Frenchness of Martinique.

In an earlier segment of the show, this internal contradiction of the republican model is dramatized during a now famous verbal confrontation opposing Christophe Martet, president of ACT UP-Paris at the time, and Culture Minister Philippe Douste-Blazy, representing the government. Martet, a public figure who identifies himself as a gay man with AIDS, sits next to his lover François as a vivid example of what it means for a same-sex couple to be deprived of legal status. In contrast with nearly everyone who has spoken before him, François insists on the fact that he is speaking as more than just an individual when he says, visibly moved: "I, as a gay man, living with Christophe, have no legal rights" ["Moi, en tant qu'homosexuel, vivant avec Christophe, je n'ai aucun droit légalement"]. Although many *individual* gays and lesbians disagreed, Martet and François were in effect the spokespersons of the gay *community* that night. In accordance with ACT UP's goal, it was as gay men that they went on to address the concern of other communities as well.

One reason for ACT UP's anger, Martet explains, is the continuing illegal deportations of people with HIV and AIDS to countries where they cannot receive adequate medical care. Martet gives the example of Marie-Louise, an undocumented immigrant from what was then Zaire. Marie-Louise is HIV-positive and her son has AIDS. Yet, both would have been deported back to Zaire if members of ACT UP and Sol En Si (Solidarité Enfants Sida, an organization dealing with children with HIV and AIDS) hadn't prevented the plane from taking off. And Martet asks: "Will France finally live up to human rights?" ["Est-ce que, enfin, la France va être digne [des?] droits de l'homme?"]. Finally, after attacking the government for neglecting prisons, refusing to legalize same-sex couples, and ignoring the DOM-TOM, a furious Martet storms off of the set, asking: "What kind of a shitty country is this?" ["C'est quoi, ce pays de merde?"]. To which Douste-Blazy replies: "To begin with, you shouldn't say such a thing. It's not right" ["D'abord il faut pas dire une chose comme ça. C'est pas bien"]. Needless to say, the event made national headlines, and ACT UP was widely held responsible not only for the poor results of the *Sidaction*, but also for jeopardizing the new and fragile sympathy enjoyed by gays and lesbians in times of hardship.[18]

Yet, Martet asked a crucial question. Obviously the issue is not, as the minister feigned to believe, to find out whether France is a shitty country. Like any other country, it is and it isn't. What is important, though, is to ask what *kind* of country it is. The story of Marie-Louise is especially significant in that respect, not so much because it shows France in an unflattering light, but mostly because it connects AIDS to the issue of immigration, which, as I discussed earlier, is where the Republic's core values are being tested and debated. The *Sidaction*, however, was not meant to be a democratic debate on the defining values of French society—quite the contrary. Dominant AIDS discourse in France is intended to replicate and reinforce the political and ethical values of the Republic, and the *Sidaction*'s purpose is to provide the nation with the opportunity to perform this ideal of Frenchness as enlightened goodness. The show's narrative of national unity could not but be disrupted by the story of Marie-Louise, the undocumented, African, HIV-positive mother of a child with AIDS, who was to be expelled in the name of the Republic. Moreover, Martet also reminded the viewers that little children are not typical PWAs, and that all the generous gifts would go to undocumented immigrants, gay men without rights, drug users, prison inmates, transsexuals, and even undocumented transsexuals. In effect, Martet's list offered a counter-narrative to the opening segment that presented those affected exclusively as white and straight. So the *Sidaction* was indeed a failure, but not only because it didn't collect the expected amount of money. It failed as a plebiscite because, thanks to a couple of angry queers, it could not quietly reconstruct the ideal Frenchness embodied by republican values.

The rhetoric of consensus does not so much seek to convince opponents to change their mind as it tries to silence them, or expel them toward the outer limits of the group performed by that rhetoric. In the debate on immigration, for example, Jean-Marie Le Pen's Front National and Islamic fundamentalists are both defined as evil and un-French; in dominant AIDS discourse, it is also the case for anything that can be labelled as identity politics. Consider for instance the rhetorical use of sick children. Because they are able to inspire universal compassion, children appear much more often in AIDS discourse than they do in AIDS statistics. As a result of this universalization, any dissenting voice is automatically defined as evil. When Martet angrily reminded viewers that for 600 cluding ACT UP-Paris, and other personalities, groups, and unions. It defined itself as the "real Left," challenging the "official Left." Although the alliance was formed to foreground certain issues in the specific context of the elections, it is tempting to read its name as a speech act transforming a republican Left into a democratic one, and eventually affecting the way France conceives itself and foresees its future. Truly, there is no choice. To the extent that the republican model of universal integration caused AIDS to spread the way it did, it must be altered. If it isn't it will only repeat and reinforce the exclusionary practices that are to blame for the deaths of tens of thousands of people.

Notes

Bibliography

Index

Introduction: Where Does AIDS Come from?

1. On the appropriation of these genres in dominant AIDS discourses, see Judith Williamson, "Every Virus Tells a Story." I discuss all these narrative and metaphorical constructions of AIDS in a more exhaustive fashion in chapter 4, where the reader will find a more complete listing of citations on these topics. On war and military metaphors specifically, Susan Sontag's *Illness as Metaphor* and *AIDS and Its Metaphors,* as well as numerous refutations, are also addressed in that chapter.

2. One of the best and most influential discussions of that aspect of the metaphoricity of AIDS discourses is to be found in Paula A. Treichler, "AIDS, Homophobia, and Biomedical Discourse." Again, I refer the reader to chapter 4 of this book.

3. See Garabed Eknoyan and Byron A. Eknoyan, "Medicine and the Case of Emile Zola," 104, and Robert A. Nye, "Degeneration and the Medical Model of Cultural Crisis in the French *Belle Epoque,*" 21.

4. Haraway, *Crystals, Fabrics, and Fields,* 9.

5. For Aristotle both terms of a metaphor must be reversible for the metaphor to work; if A is like B, then B is like A. See *The Art of Rhetoric.*

6. I shall elaborate more on this idea in chapter 1.

7. From *Models and Analogies in Science,* quoted by Haraway, 10.

8. See Georges Canguilhem, *The Normal and the Pathological.*

9. One could argue that Genet's work was not as well known to the mainstream public as Guibert's was. This is due, I think, to the differences in their respective cultural and historical contexts. Genet's fame was established at a time when the media did not have the reach they now have. In a word, Genet became famous before television. What would have happened if he had appeared on the scene in the early 1990s is impossible to know, of course, but it is interesting to notice that in his hugely successful novel and film *Les nuits fauves,* Cyril Collard made ample use of Genet, both intertextually and explicitly, to construct a self-image of rebellion that was quickly recuperated by mainstream as well as subaltern cultures.

10. Author-actor-director Cyril Collard is another example. And it is hard not to think of Arthur Rimbaud, also canonical as well as a figure of rebellion, whose portrait is often spray-painted on the walls of French cities. And although he is not a French author, Truman Capote comes to mind too. His lascivious pose in the photograph on the back of his first novel, *Other Voices, Other Rooms,* became as notorious as the book itself. The fact that

Genet, Guibert, Rimbaud, and Capote, all of them cult figures, were open homosexuals for whom the closet seemed never to have existed certainly has a lot to do with their popular constructions as objects of both desire and fear, and it should be the object of a specific study. (The Romantics, of course, had already discovered how author portraits could increase book sales, if the author happened to be attractive.)

Chapter 1. Degeneracy and Inversion

1. See, in particular, Sander Gilman's *The Jew's Body* and *Difference and Pathology*, Edward Chamberlin and Gilman, eds., *Degeneration*, and George L. Mosse's *Nationalism and Sexuality*. For both Gilman and Mosse, homosexuality and Jewishness are merely avatars of otherness in general.

2. Antony Copley, *Sexual Moralities in France, 1780–1980*, 148.

3. All translations are mine unless signaled by a page number after the English version.

4. See Daniel Pick, *Faces of Degeneration*, 50.

5. I am borrowing the expression "dark side" from Chamberlin and Gilman, eds., *Degeneration*.

6. Borie, *Mythologies de l'hérédité au XIXème siècle*, 11.

7. See Pick: "*Dégénérescence* had a hidden narrative development—a genesis, a law of progress, and a denouement. Complete idiocy, sterility and death were the end points in a slow accumulation of morbidity across generations" (51).

8. See John H. Smith, "Abulia: Sexuality and Diseases of the Will in the Late Nineteenth Century," and Robert A. Nye, *Crime, Madness, and Politics in Modern France*.

9. See my introduction.

10. Cohen, "Legislating the Norm," 171. See also Dominique Fernandez, *Le rapt de Ganymède*, 62; David F. Greenberg, *The Construction of Homosexuality*, 409; and Jonathan Ned Katz, *The Invention of Heterosexuality*.

11. If the following discussion deals solely with male homosexuality this is not an arbitrary choice on my part. Female homosexuality, and indeed all female sexuality, occupies only a marginal position in nineteenth-century medical literature. As Georges Lanteri-Laura rightly explains in his *Lecture des perversions: histoire de leur appropriation médicale*: "It is mainly about male homosexuality since, in all these works of science, antifeminism is compulsory, and women appear more as objects to provide sexual pleasure than subjects of that pleasure" ["Il s'agit surtout de l'homosexualité masculine, car, dans tous ces travaux de science, l'antiféminisme est de rigueur, et la femme apparaît plus à titre d'objet qui fait jouir que de sujet qui jouit" (42 n. 13)]. Moreover, as I have already mentioned, women were then considered almost pathological by definition. The fact that some might be lesbians hardly made any difference since giving in to unnatural sexual impulses betrayed the absence of a strong will, and a strong will, as we have seen, was supposed to be a healthy male characteristic.

12. For Copley, "in Victorian thinking this [masturbation] was tantamount to proof of homosexuality" (106).

13. See, for example, Copley, but also Dominique Fernandez, *Le rapt de Ganymède*.

14. The debate around a potential genetic origin of sexual orientation found a new life in the aftermath of Simon LeVay's book *The Sexual Brain*, and is now a crucial element in the various discourses on civil rights for gay, lesbian, and transgendered people.

15. As Copley has shown, the distinction between *perversion* and *perversité* is central in the works of many French forensic scientists such as H. Legludic, Léon Thoinot, and Zola's friend Georges Saint-Paul [Dr. Laupts].

16. Gilman, "Sexology, Psychoanalysis, and Degeneration," 88.

17. Mosse, *Nationalism and Sexuality,* 24.

18. See, in particular, Robert A. Nye, *Crime, Madness, and Politics*, 134–35, and André Armengaud, *La population française au XIXème siècle.* Between the years 1872 and 1911 the French population increased at a rate inferior by one third to that of the years 1821–1846.

19. This being said, the signifiers "homosexual," "invert," "effeminate," or "degenerate" did serve to describe the sexuality of the Other. Colonized populations, particularly in North Africa and Indochina, were seen as propagating homosexuality. Zola's friend Dr. Georges Saint-Paul [Dr. Laupts] is a good example. His case studies warn his readers of the dangers of sexual contacts with peoples of the Orient, where the boundaries between masculine and feminine are not so clearly defined. Surprisingly, homosexuality was also often described as a German disease, as if to temper the positive image of the victor as a model of fertility. In fact, homosexuality seems to have been the perfect label to apply to all sorts of political enemies. On the home front, political "agitators" were described as effeminate, and devirilized by feminism (see William Hirsch, *Genius and Degeneration*). Crowds, and particularly rioting urban crowds, were said to be composed of pederasts and hysterical women. (The French expression *hystérie collective,* to describe the irrational behavior of masses, endures to this day.) In Gustave Le Bon's *Psychologie des foules* (1895), a crowd's collective behavior is coded as feminine, and its leaders as effeminate.

20. See Nordau, *Degeneration*.

21. Kaempfer, *Emile Zola,* 178.

22. We can see today the logical continuation of this displacement: the *effet de réel* being replaced by what we could term an *effet de réalisme,* as in televison "reality shows." See Roland Barthes, "L'effet de réel," in *Littérature et réalité,* 81–90.

Chapter 2. Gender Indecision and Cultural Anxiety

1. Several critics have already debated the issue. See, for example, Y. Malinas, *Zola et les hérédités imaginaires;* Malinas shows that Zola's theses may not be as outlandish as previously assumed, and that in fact they seem to point rather reasonably toward the evolution of genetics.

2. By metaphor I mean all analogical structures in the widest sense, thus following more or less faithfully the definition of metaphors given by Jean Ricardou in *Problèmes du nouveau roman*. Ricardou writes that he "will call metaphors all figures constructed on three elements: the *comparé*, the *comparant*, the common point authorizing (or produced by) the comparison, that is to say, metaphors, similes, figurative meanings" ["seront appelées métaphores toutes figures construites sur trois éléments: le comparé, le comparant, le point commun autorisant (ou issu de) la comparaison, c'est-à-dire les métaphores, les comparaisons, les sens figurés" (134)]. For the concept of "generative metaphor" I will also use the definition Ricardou gives in *Le nouveau roman,* in which he calls "generative metaphor" (métaphore génératrice) a metaphor that generates a fiction, such as in La Fontaine's fables (280).

3. See, for example, David Baguley's interesting analysis in "Le récit de guerre."

4. For quotations in English, I use the 1968 translation, *The Debacle,* unless otherwise indicated. For quotations in French, I use the volume from the Gallimard edition of *Les Rougon-Macquart.*

5. Although Zola's involvement in the Dreyfus affair as well as his numerous writings on the topic of Jews amply prove that he was not an anti-Semite, it shouldn't come as a surprise to find traces of anti-Semitism in his fictional writings. In *L'argent,* the volume of the Rougon-Macquart series immediately preceding *La débâcle* and inspired by the crash of the Catholic bank Union Générale, Zola had already used the old stereotype associating Jews with money and the world of high finance.

6. On the image of the *Ostjuden* I send the reader to Sander Gilman's abundant work.

7. In her excellent study of nineteenth-century narratives of hysteria, Beizer observes how, in a discourse that pathologizes femininity, uncontrolled and exaggerated speech in women mirrors their excessive flow of bodily secretions. Beizer writes: "The hysteria doctors often stress that even normal women (that is, protohysterics) secrete tears, sweat, gastric juices, bile, and urine more quickly and in greater abundance than do men. They are also prone to an analogous flow of chatter, gossip, exaggerations, and lies" (*Ventriloquized Bodies,* 191). In chapter 5 I return to the role of gossip and rumors in the elaboration of knowledge from the margins of power.

8. From *Nouvelle campagne,* quoted by Helen Beatrice Rufener, *Biography of a War Novel,* 93.

9. Beizer, "The Body in Question," 51. See also *Ventriloquized Bodies.*

10. Zola, *L'atelier de Zola,* ed. Martin Kanes, 220–21. In a conversation with the Goncourt brothers, Zola hinted that he, too, might have had some homosexual experience while in high school in Aix. See Graham King, *Garden of Zola,* 3.

11. Zola, *L'atelier de Zola,* 224–25.

12. Dr. Laupts, [Georges Saint-Paul], *L'homosexualité et les types homosexuels.* Saint-Paul gave the manuscript the title "Novel of a Born Invert" ["Journal d'un inverti-né" (431)].

13. John Lapp, "The Watcher Betrayed and the Fatal Woman," 282. For a more detailed discussion of the *petit crevé,* see Robert Lethbridge, "Zola," and Antoine Com-

pagnon, "Zola dans la décadence." About Zola's sexual molestation at the age of five by a twelve-year-old Algerian servant named Mustapha, see Lapp, "The Watcher Betrayed and the Fatal Woman," and Karl Rosen, "Emile Zola and Homosexuality," as well as many biographies. Many critics and biographers want to read in this episode the origin of Zola's hatred of homosexuality. Such endeavors, needless to say, are eminently suspect.

14. See Maurice Descotes, "Le personnage de Napoléon III dans *Les Rougon-Macquart.*"

15. On the structural role of King William's position during the battle, see David Baguley, "Le récit de guerre."

16. To get an idea of how such stereotypical portrayals have endured almost unchanged for more than a hundred years, a dossier on homosexuality published by *L'événement du jeudi* (3–9 December 1992) provides edifying reading. The dossier is entitled "La tragédie homosexuelle" but it is never really clear whether the "tragedy" in question is AIDS or homosexuality itself. The reporter, a liberal heterosexual woman, is describing the inside of a Parisian gay bar:

> At the bar, some white, waxy faces are dripping with sweat; the make-up leaves traces. Sometimes, their skin looks like a veil, stretched over the bones. Thinning hair, deep, feverish gazes. They order a drink with the light gesture of a queen of the night, and hold their cigarettes with the tips of their fingers, like women do. In some gazes, the offer is brutally and immediately there. (my translation)

> [Au bar, quelques visages blancs, cireux, luisent de sueur; les fonds de teint laissent des traces. Certains ont la peau comme un voile, tendue sur les os. Cheveux clairsemés, regard enfoncé, fiévreux. Ils commandent un verre d'un geste léger de belle de nuit et tiennent leur cigarette au bout des doigts, comme une femme. Dans certains regards, la demande est là, brutale, immédiate. (73)]

17. See Burton Pike, *The Image of the City in Modern Literature.*

18. See Henri Mitterand's dossier on Zola's notes (Zola, *Les Rougon-Macquart,* vol. 5, 1379).

19. See Naomi Schor, *Zola's Crowds.*

20. See Serres's analysis (*Feux et signaux de brume*) on the metaphor of the flow in *La débâcle,* which differs from mine; see also Beizer's analysis of the menstrual metaphor in "The Body in Question."

21. Interestingly enough, the most endearing couples in the Rougon-Macquart cycle often do not represent the heterosexual ideal of procreation so central to Zola's essays and articles. See for instance Carol Colatrella's excellent analysis of Miette and Sylvère in *La fortune des Rougon,* the opening novel of the cycle ("Representing Liberty"). Colatrella shows how Miette, in order to represent liberty, must be a virgin; yet, Zola must have her killed since only motherhood can save the nation. In "Androgyny and Morality in *Germinal,*" Claudia Moscovici studies the ambiguous relationship between a masculine Catherine Maheu and a feminized Etienne Lantier, another story of ideal but impossible

love. On the lesbian love affair between Nana and Satin, see Schor, *Zola's Crowds*. Also on *Nana*, but with wider implications concerning Zola's inability to stick to his avowed project, see Sandy Petrey, "Anna-Nana-Nana."

22. See Eve Kosofsky Sedgwick, *Between Men*.

23. David Baguley, "Le récit de guerre."

24. In his article "La république de *La débâcle*," Sandy Petrey rightly remarks that "ordinarily, it is not madmen who explain the value of reason" ["Ce ne sont pas d'ordinaire les fous qui expliquent la valeur de la raison" (94)]. Petrey reads this as a general tendency in the novel not to represent what it is supposed to preach, such as the Republic, for example. In the case of Maurice, we could even conclude that Zola praises in fact the exact opposite of what he preaches.

25. Jean will return in *Le docteur Pascal*. Back to the Plassans area of his roots, Jean will marry a phenomenally fertile peasant woman, "one of these cases of pullulating fecundity which don't give mothers enough time to breast-feed their little ones" ["un de ces cas de fécondité pullulante qui ne laissent pas aux mères le temps d'allaiter leurs petits" (*Les Rougon-Macquart*, vol. 5, 1017)]. Together they represent the regeneration of the community, in direct opposition to little Charles, the vicious, perverse, effeminate *fin de race*, who will slowly bleed to death. The heterosexual order is restored, and Zola can conclude: "The work was good, when there was a child at the end of love" ["L'oeuvre était bonne, quand il y avait l'enfant, au bout de l'amour" (1218)].

Chapter 3. Reclaiming Disease and Infection

1. For more specific information on that period, see Albert Dichy and Pascal Fouché, *Jean Genet: essai de chronologie, 1910–1944*; Jean-Bernard Moraly, *Jean Genet: la vie écrite*; and Edmund White, *Genet: A Biography*.

2. See chapter 1.

3. See White, "The Novelist Thief."

4. As will become clearer, I am using Gilles Deleuze and Félix Guattari's term "deterritorialization" with a more literal meaning too. See *L'anti-Oedipe*.

5. From *The American Heritage Dictionary of the English Language*. New York: American Heritage Publishing, 1973.

6. See the version of *Pompes funèbres* in the Biblos collection (1993), not the one included by Gallimard in Genet's complete works.

7. See Bourdieu, *The Rules of Art*.

8. To be frank, it had always been rather explicit. For example, the very first sentence of Genet's very first novel, *Notre-Dame-des-fleurs* (*Our Lady of the Flowers*) includes a now famous antagonistic *vous*, addressed to the readers and situating Genet's voice on the side of crime. Talking about the picture of a notorious murderer soon to be sent to the guillotine, Genet writes: "Weidmann appeared before you in a five o'clock edition . . . " (61) ["Weidmann vous apparut dans une édition de cinq heures . . . " (10)]. In fact, Genet's

publishers initially thought that the *vous* was a spelling mistake, and that Genet really meant to write *nous*.

9. As we have seen in previous chapters, these three terms are often synonymous in discourses emanating from late-nineteenth-century medical discourse.

10. The word *état* indicates that Genet may also be saying something about the nation-state being infected.

11. The term *pestiféré* is still used to describe someone with whom contact is perceived to be dangerous, but the virulence of the plague indicates a foretaste of death rather than a state of exclusion.

12. I use the masculine since, in the text, the metaphor applies only to men.

13. I will return to Genet's use of the medieval intertext later in this chapter.

14. Commenting on his earlier writings, Genet writes in *Journal du voleur:*

[I]f I examine my work, I now perceive in it, patiently pursued, a will to rehabilitate persons, objects and feelings reputedly vile. Naming them with words that usually designate what is noble was perhaps childish and somewhat facile. . . . but I would not have done so were it not that, within me, those objects, those feelings (treason, theft, cowardice, fear), called for the qualifier generally reserved—by you—for their opposites. (109)

[[S]i j'examine ce que j'écrivis j'y distingue aujourd'hui, patiemment poursuivie, une volonté de réhabilitation des êtres, des objets, des sentiments réputés vils. De les avoir nommés avec les mots qui d'habitude désignent la noblesse, c'était peut-être enfantin, facile. . . . mais je ne l'eusse pas fait si, en moi-même, ces objets, ces sentiments (la trahison, le vol, la lâcheté, la peur) n'eussent appelé le qualificatif réservé d'habitude et par vous à leurs contraires. (115)]

15. In chapter 5 I develop the idea that gossip and rumors, because they have an epidemic structure, can be positively reclaimed to disseminate decentered discourses of knowledge in order to form, serve, and enable marginalized communities.

16. See Sontag, *Illness as Metaphor,* for a more thorough discussion of this type of rhetorical displacement. See also my next chapter for a discussion of this issue in the specific context of AIDS.

17. We have known for a while now that much of the information Genet provided about his life was in fact fabricated. See the biographies mentioned in note 1, as well as Michael Sheringham's essay "Narration and Experience in Genet's *Journal du voleur*" for a discussion of the autobiographical issues in this text.

18. In *The Vision of Jean Genet,* Richard N. Coe bases his entire analysis of Genet's work (at least up until the 1960s, since his study was written in 1968) on what he calls "the most characteristic of all Genet's symbols" (25). Situating his own study within a strict Sartrean framework, Coe writes: "Thus the fusion of mirror-opposites, of positive and negative, is gradually resolved, in Genet's later works, into a kind of ferocious and deliberately repulsive Hegelian dialectic: thesis, antithesis and synthesis" (24). This reading,

however, adds little to Sartre's study and fails to account for the deconstructionist dimension of Genet's work. Frieda Ekotto's idea that, for Genet, mutually exclusive terms are engaged in a process of permanent negotiation, is much more accurate and fruitful (*L'écriture carcérale et le discours juridique chez Jean Genet et Roger Knobelspiess*).

19. I want to thank Yvon Bonnet for telling me about this term.

20. See Chambers, *Room for Maneuver,* for a discussion of (internal) oppositionality versus (external) resistance. Genet's politics, like everything else about him, are not easy to classify in that respect, since he seemed, throughout his life, to advocate both strategies in order to effect social change.

21. While it primarily owes a debt to Julia Kristeva, Mary Douglas, and Georges Bataille, my reading of Genet also incorporates definitions of the terms "abject" and "abjection" similar to the ones given by Butler in *Bodies That Matter.* I find such definitions to be particularly productive when dealing with *Journal du voleur.* Butler writes:

> The abject designates here precisely those "unlivable" and "uninhabitable" zones of social life which are nevertheless densely populated by those who do not enjoy the status of the subject, but whose living under the sign of the "unlivable" is required to circumscribe the domain of the subject. . . . In this sense, then, the subject is constituted through the force of exclusion and abjection, one which produces a constitutive outside to the subject, an abjected outside, which is, after all, "inside" the subject as its own founding repudiation. (3)

22. In *Saint Genet,* Sartre gives us an excellent analysis of a lie based on a true (?) episode in Genet's life. Genet managed to steal a rare and precious book by sending the clerk to get another book that he didn't really want. The lie triggered a series of actions on the part of the clerk, but, Sartre writes:

> The fact is that he is not acting, he is dancing: he goes to get *for nothing* a book that nobody wants to buy; his eagerness, his smile, which ordinarily aim at charming customers, are mere pantomime since there are no customers in the shop but only a thief who cannot be charmed. And the result of this pantomime is a denial of the real world to the advantage of a universe of pure appearance. (281; original emphasis)

> [Or il n'agit pas, il danse: il va chercher *pour rien* un livre que nul ne veut acheter; son empressement, son sourire qui visent ordinairement à séduire la clientèle sont de simples pantomimes, puisqu'il n'y a pas de clients au magasin mais seulement un voleur qui ne peut être séduit. Et cette pantomime a pour résultat de nier le monde vrai au profit d'un univers de pure apparence. (316; original emphasis)]

23. In his essay "L'abjection et les formes misérables," Bataille underscores the fragility of the boundary and "the inability to assume forcefully enough the imperative act of exclusion of abject things" ["l'incapacité d'assumer avec une force suffisante l'acte impératif d'exclusion des choses abjectes" (*Oeuvres complètes,* vol. 12, 219)]. In that essay, he de-

fines abject things as "objects of the imperative act of exclusion" ["objets de l'acte impératif d'exclusion" (220)].

24. Again, see Sartre's analysis quoted in note 22.

25. White's biography tells us that Genet was actually in contact with German members of the resistance movement against Hitler.

26. Genet capitalizes on an old Western tradition associating the sea with plagues and other epidemics. Here, the ocean also recalls the image of the ship of fools (analyzed by Michel Foucault in *Madness and Civilization*).

27. In *Querelle de Brest* Genet tells the story of Querelle, a handsome sailor and murderer. The novel opens with another of Genet's famous sentences: "The notion of murder often brings to mind the notion of sea and sailors" (3) ["L'idée de meurtre évoque souvent l'idée de mer, de marins" (173)]. And, emphasizing that he is more interested in myths than in reality, he adds: "If one considers that seaports are the scene of frequent crimes, the association seems self-explanatory; but there are numerous stories from which we learn that the murderer was a man of the sea—either a real one, or a fake one—and if the latter is the case, the crime will be even more closely connected to the sea" (3) ["Si les ports sont le théâtre répété de crimes, l'explication en est facile que nous n'entreprendrons pas, mais nombreuses sont les chroniques où l'on apprend que l'assassin était un navigateur, faux ou vrai et s'il est faux le crime en a de plus étroits rapports avec la mer" (173)].

28. If I were writing in French, I would use the partitive *du* in that sentence: *du positif et du négatif, de l'intérieur et de l'extérieur, du sujet et de l'objet.*

29. Hocquenghem observes that in hetero-capitalist societies, "The only acceptable form of homosexual temporality is that which is directed towards the past" (*Homosexual Desire*, 93–94).

30. See Bataille's chapter on Genet's "failure" in *Literature and Evil.*

31. In fact, Genet himself described his "passage" from literature to politics as one of these border crossings, as if going from one world to another, while acknowledging the theoretical impossibility of separating the two. In a 1983 interview with Rüdiger Wischenbart and Layla Shahid Barrada published by the *Revue d'études palestiniennes,* he described his move toward the Black Panthers and the Palestinians as follows: "I was acting in terms of the real world and no longer in terms of the grammatical world. Insofar as one sees the real world and the world of dreams as opposites. Of course, if one carries the analysis further, one knows full well that dreaming is also a part of the real world" ["j'agissais en fonction du monde réel et plus en fonction du monde grammatical. Dans la mesure où on oppose le monde réel au monde de la rêverie. Bien sûr, si on pousse plus loin l'analyse, on sait bien que la rêverie appartient aussi au monde réel" (*Oeuvres complètes,* vol. 6, 277)]. Genet's political writings make up the sixth volume of his *Oeuvres complètes,* under the title *L'ennemi déclaré.* For an analysis of that dimension of Genet's work, see Hadrien Laroche, *Le dernier Genet,* in which the author likens Genet's move from literature to politics and back to crossing the strait of Gibraltar twice. And in a description that seems to echo Genet's peregrinations in *Journal du voleur,* Laroche writes:

"Between the two passages of the strait . . . he can be seen in Chicago, he can be seen in Jordan, he makes the trips to Strasbourg and Chartres. He meets with parties and movements and their members: the Black Panthers in the United States, the Red Army Fraction in Germany, the Palestinians in the Middle East" ["Entre les deux traversées du détroit . . . [o]n le voit à Chicago, on le voit en Jordanie, il se déplace à Strasbourg ou à Chartres. Il rencontre des partis, des mouvements, les hommes qui les composent: Panthères noires aux Etats-Unis, Fraction Armée rouge en Allemagne, Palestiniens au Moyen-Orient" (8)].

Chapter 4. A Cultural History of AIDS Discourse

1. Douglas Crimp, "AIDS: Cultural Analysis, Cultural Activism," 3; Paula A. Treichler, "AIDS, Homophobia, and Biomedical Discourse," 31; Simon Watney, *Policing Desire*, 9. Crimp, Treichler, and Watney, as well as Cindy Patton, Jeffrey Weeks, and a few other Anglo-American critics, produced the first interesting analyses of AIDS discourses in the early and mid-1980s. In France, however, and despite the fact that it was—and still is—the Western nation most affected by AIDS after the United States, it took a long time for such politically oriented criticism to come out. Many reasons have been proposed to explain why France was so slow to respond to the epidemic in general, from cultural taboos about sexuality and disease to the collapse of gay and lesbian activism following François Mitterrand's first election to the presidency. While these factors undoubtedly played a part, it should also be added that the universalist republican model structuring modern French society does not recognize the presence of communities in its midst, therefore making it very difficult for the French to realize how the AIDS epidemic in the West has primarily affected marginalized communities. I shall return to this issue in greater detail in the conclusion of this book. On this topic, see also Frank Arnal, *Résister ou disparaître?*; Fabienne Worth, "Le sacré et le sida"; Yves Roussel, "Le mouvement homosexuel français face aux stratégies identitaires"; and Claude Deslhiat, "L'aveuglement des années 1982–1985 et ses causes." In all fairness, Frédéric Martel's much publicized study *Le rose et le noir* should also be mentioned, despite its obvious lack of academic rigor and its outlandish claim that the gay community was the main culprit for early denials of AIDS in France. Martel's book, too, will be dealt with in the conclusion.

2. Marsan, *La vie blessée*, 19.

3. In the early years of the epidemic, the prevailing attitude in France consisted of avoiding panic. AIDS, we were told, was just a disease and should be treated as such, that is, rationally and scientifically. There should be no finger-pointing, no scapegoating, and no apocalytic discourse about the approaching millennium. That, in a nutshell, was *dé-dramatisation*. Today, it has become clear to most participants in the public discourse of AIDS that it was only blindness and denial. I would add that it was also an expression of French anti-Americanism. The hysterical reactions described above were generally at-

tributed to the United States. France—socialist France, at the time—could in turn construct itself once more as the reliable locus of enlightenment, reason, and humanist values.

4. See chapters 1 and 2.

5. Susan Sontag, *Illness as Metaphor* and *AIDS and Its Metaphors;* Sander L. Gilman, *Disease and Representation* and other works.

6. See chapter 1.

7. I am referring here, for example, to the work of Luc Montagnier, whose team first discovered HIV, and who has been investigating the possible role of cofactors in the development of AIDS. I am not alluding to those who claim that HIV is not in any way connected to AIDS and who often promote a thinly veiled homophobic agenda.

8. See John Nguyet Erni, *Unstable Frontiers.*

9. For more on early PWA mobilization, see Max Navarre, "Fighting the Victim Label" and "PWA Coalition Portfolio"; see also ACT UP-Paris, *Le sida.*

10. See in particular Christopher C. Taylor, "AIDS and the Pathogenesis of Metaphor."

11. Watney, "Taking Liberties," 37.

12. For another analysis of this issue in Jean Genet's *Journal du voleur,* see chapter 3.

13. Williamson, "Every Virus Tells a Story."

14. Crimp, "How to Have Promiscuity in an Epidemic," 244–45; Barthes, *Le degré zéro de l'écriture,* 44–45.

15. Watney, *Policing Desire,* 22–23.

16. I did not mention children, hemophiliacs, and people who received blood transfusions, that is, the so-called innocent victims of AIDS. It is not a coincidence if the earliest efforts to fight the epidemic were directed at these categories. With the appearance of expensive new drugs known as protease inhibitors, the economic disparities between different categories of people with AIDS appeared more shocking than ever, as it became perfectly clear to everyone that poor Africans, for example, were at great risk of never benefiting from these new treatments unless something was done to challenge the power of the pharmaceutical industry.

17. In France in the late 1990s, 40 percent of AIDS cases were found among gay men, and another 40 percent among IV drug users.

18. Watney, "Representing AIDS"; Grover, "Constitutional Symptoms"; see also Brian Patton, "Cell Wars"; and Michael S. Sherry, "The Language of War in AIDS Discourse." In *Sain[t]s et saufs,* Alain Ménil defends a position very similar to Sontag's, but for him, the danger lies less in using metaphors to talk about a disease than in considering the disease itself as metaphor because, as he concludes, "if the disease in question is only a metaphor, then one will only seek to treat that for which it is a metaphor" ["si la maladie en question n'est qu'une métaphore, c'est à traiter ce dont elle est la métaphore qu'il faut travailler" (212)].

19. In an interview given to the French gay magazine *Ex aequo* in 1997, Alain Finkielkraut still claimed the opposite, as he launched into a larger homophobic attack against Gay Pride parades and the gay community as a whole. He states:

In the early years, when research wasn't going anywhere, we were told that if this disease didn't concern homosexuals, a cure would have been found. What happened is the exact opposite. Advances in AIDS research have been incomparably faster than they have in cancer research, and social awareness has been far more important. One must have the courage to say that the fact that AIDS is a disease that spread among homosexuals hasn't delayed anything at all.

[Pendant les années où la recherche piétinait, on nous disait que si cette maladie ne visait pas les homosexuels, on aurait trouvé des remèdes. C'est exactement le contraire qui s'est produit. Les progrès de la recherche sur le sida ont été incomparablement plus rapides que les progrès de la recherche sur le cancer, et la mobilisation sociale beaucoup plus importante. Il faut avoir le courage de dire que le fait que le sida soit une maladie répandue parmi les homosexuels n'a rien retardé du tout. (44)]

What Finkielkraut fails to see, of course, is that there was no real national awareness of AIDS, no "mobilisation sociale," until the state-sanctioned contamination of "innocent" hemophiliacs was exposed in 1991, and that research and societal responses to AIDS began to accelerate in large part because of gay activism, mostly from the ranks of Aides and ACT UP-Paris. In a fashion typical of anti-politically-correct rhetoric, the "courage" Finkielkraut speaks of is a fictional construct whose sole, self-promoting purpose is for Finkielkraut himself to embody it. More on this in my conclusion.

20. Louis Pauwels, "Le monôme des zombis," *Le Figaro Magazine*, 6 Dec. 1986. Quoted by Rieusset-Lemarié, *Une fin de siècle épidémique*, 140.

21. In "Right On, Girlfriend!" Douglas Crimp talks about "a new kind of indifference, an indifference that has been called the 'normalization of AIDS'" (5).

22. See chapters 1 and 2.

23. In fact, it had never really disappeared and was actually reinforced with the biomedical construction of the Other as intrinsically sick.

24. Obviously I am not implying that AIDS is the only factor explaining the resurgence of xenophobia and nationalisms in the West; but it has certainly played a part in it, first because it is an epidemic and epidemics have a long history of generating exclusion and scapegoating, and second because AIDS was initially constructed as the disease of the Other.

25. For the best analysis of this dual determination of AIDS and its early periodization, see *Inventing AIDS*, in which Cindy Patton argues that, because AIDS was first conceptualized within the field of immunology (as a collapse of the immune system) and then within that of virology (as a transmissible disease), two different sets of metaphors and politics developed consecutively. I discuss these issues in the introduction.

26. "It seems logical that the political figure in France who represents the most extreme nativist, racist views, Jean-Marie Le Pen, has attempted a strategy of fomenting fear of this new alien peril, insisting that AIDS is not just infectious but contagious, and call-

ing for mandatory nationwide testing and the quarantine of everyone carrying the virus" (Sontag, *AIDS and Its Metaphors*, 150). It would be a mistake to think that, because Le Pen represents such an extreme political position, excessive importance shouldn't be given to his views, or that, precisely because they come from him, such words are guaranteed never to enter mainstream public discourse. In fact, the senate, a traditional stronghold of conservatism, tried on several occasions to pass legislation criminalizing homosexuality or mandating HIV testing.

27. Bachelot describes people with HIV or AIDS as extraterrestrials, terrorists, viral time bombs, and so on (Tort, "Du fascisme sanitaire," 44).

28. For more on the various reactions to Bachelot's statements, see *SIDA'venture: SIDA, éthique, discriminations*. On the Front National's positions on AIDS see Pierre Mathiot, "Le sida dans la stratégie et la rhétorique du Front national."

29. On the military allegory and the idea of borders see Martine Delvaux's reading of Alain Emmanuel Dreuilhe's AIDS journal *Corps à corps* in "Des corps et des frontières."

30. Michael Lynch, "Living with Kaposi's," *Body Politic* 88 (Nov. 1982), quoted in Treichler, "AIDS, Homophobia, and Biomedical Discourse," 40.

31. Christopher Craft, "'Kiss me with those red lips.'"

32. See chapter 1.

33. Richard Dyer, "Children of the Night."

34. In "Undead," Ellis Hanson draws on Ernest Jones's *On the Nightmare* and the unconscious link between blood and semen: "Ernest Jones informs us that anal eroticism and infantile perversion, virtues generally reserved for homosexuals, are at the core of the necrophilous vampire myth. Then, of course, there is Jones's further equation of semen with blood in the unconscious, a theory which has the unfortunate consequence of rendering every cocksucker into a kind of bloodsucker" (328).

35. I do not claim as my own the idea that the figure of Oscar Wilde's Dorian Gray can be used to read some representations of visibly marked PWAs. It may be found in many essays, including the ones by Watney, Hanson, Dyer, and Meyer, mentioned earlier, and Jeff Nunokawa, "'All the Sad Young Men.'"

36. Little by little, these images have been replaced with emblems of dignity and courage designed to inspire compassion and generosity. The recent *Sidaction*, huge French fundraising TV shows, have shown us, however, that in order to receive donations it is better to exhibit the least representative "victims" of AIDS, such as children, courageous spouses of PWAs, and grandparents left to raise the kids of their dead children. Gay men are welcome if they seem unhappy about their sexuality, and IV drug users if they are going through detox hell. At any rate, all political outbursts, ACT UP style, are considered inappropriate and in poor taste. I am thinking of Christophe Martet, then president of ACT UP-Paris, who angrily confronted Philippe Douste-Blazy, former minister of health, during the 1996 *Sidaction*. For a discussion of this incident and how the *Sidaction* exemplifies dominant constructions of AIDS in France today, see the conclusion of this book. See also Ménil, *Sain[t]s et saufs*.

37. Williamson shows how HIV has become the protagonist of narratives modeled on

detective stories, for example. Treichler, in "AIDS, Homophobia, and Biomedical Discourse," sees the figure of the spy or the international terrorist as a common narrativization of HIV. The "homosexual" includes all these connotations.

38. On this issue, see my article "Intrusions."

39. Bernard Sellier, "De la difficulté de vivre," 52. See also Grover, "Visible Lesions," for similar anecdotes as well as an analysis of early representations of PWAs in the media, and Crimp, "Portraits of People with AIDS."

40. In France, Cyril Collard was one of the first celebrities to challenge the image of the weak and dying PWA. In the United States, sports celebrities like Magic Johnson or Greg Louganis had the same effect (although their self-construction and heroization were quite different from Collard's). Today, protease inhibitors and combination therapies have mostly displaced the question: The treatment seems to be working . . . but for how long?

41. A sadly comical example comes from the now-defunct Agence Française de Lutte contre le Sida (AFLS), a French government agency in charge of AIDS prevention. The AFLS produced a series of little booklets on safe sex entitled "Hommes entre eux" ("Men among themselves") directly targeting the gay community. Some brochures deal with a specific sexual practice—oral sex, S/M, and so on—some with a rather generic type of gay social life, and always in a fairly explicit fashion. Not too much ground for complaint, apparently, except that the brochures come with the warning "Réservé à un public averti." (The word *averti* can be translated both as "forewarned" and "well-informed.") The information, therefore, seems to be targeted at those who are already informed! In addition, one could also argue that the title of the series, "Men among *themselves*" as opposed to "*ourselves*," only reinforces the exclusion of the men in question. For a study on the failures of safe sex campaigns, see Cindy Patton, *Fatal Advice*.

42. For a clever, albeit problematic, deconstruction of the opposition between passivity and activism as homophobic, see Lee Edelman, "The Mirror and the Tank."

43. Grover, "Visible Lesions," 12; original emphasis.

44. In July 1997, the French governement finally authorized emergency treatments for all.

45. The distinction between innocent and guilty victims was particularly obvious in the 1990s when several states in the United States tried to pass legislation mandating that all pregnant women be tested for HIV antibodies in order to protect the life of the fetus.

46. Again, this has been a political issue with legal ramifications, as several states and countries have made it a crime to have unprotected sex when knowing that one is HIV-positive.

Chapter 5. AIDS and the Unraveling of Modernity

1. For overviews of Hervé Guibert's writings, see mostly Jean-Pierre Boulé's work, but also Henk Hillenaar, "Hervé Guibert (1955–1991)"; Ralph Sarkonak, "Traces and Shadows"; and Edmund White, "Hervé Guibert."

2. On the importance of Guibert's TV appearances and their role in his construction as a media sensation, see Boulé, "Hervé Guibert à la télévision."

3. ACT UP-Paris, *Le sida,* 176.

4. Quoted by Boulé, *Hervé Guibert,* 12.

5. Pagination for the English translation is from the Serpent's Tail edition, *To the Friend Who Did Not Save My Life.* Pagination from the French text is from the original Gallimard "Collection Blanche" edition. I will henceforth use the abbreviation *A l'ami.*

6. From Guibert, "La vie sida," 21.

7. See in particular Raymond Bellour, "Trompe-la-mort"; Jean-Pierre Boulé, introduction to the Guibert issue of *Nottingham French Studies;* Frédéric Martel, "Guibert, Koltès, Copi"; and Edmund White, "Hervé Guibert."

8. Dominique Fernandez, "La liberté, tombeau de l'inspiration," 11. This openly gay author also developed the same thesis—based on the idea that gay liberation means the end of centuries of exceptional gay creativity because oppression is necessary for there to be genius—in his book-length essay *Le rapt de Ganymède* and his AIDS novel *La gloire du paria.* For a detailed refutation of Fernandez's argument, see Ménil, *Sain[t]s et saufs.*

9. Derek Duncan, "Gestes autobiographiques," 101.

10. A notable exception would be Dreuilhe's *Corps à corps,* but it was actually written in New York, where the author had been living for a while. To a large extent, *Corps à corps* depicts a very American experience of AIDS as well as gayness.

11. An exception is Copi's play *Une visite inopportune.* In "Guibert, Koltès, Copi," Martel argues that Bernard-Marie Koltès's last plays deal with AIDS in a nonthematic way.

12. For more detailed studies, mostly based on Antonin Artaud's writings, see Isabelle Rieusset-Lemarié, *Une fin de siècle épidémique,* and Richard C. Ledes and Martin G. Koloski, "AIDS and the Ninjas."

13. There is little doubt that such cultural traditions were hypocritically essentialized to avoid addressing AIDS as a public crisis.

14. For overviews of AIDS literature in France see Martel, *Le rose et le noir;* Christopher Robinson, *Scandal in the Ink;* and David Wetsel, "The Best of Times, the Worst of Times."

15. See my article "Intrusions," and Vito Russo, *The Celluloid Closet,* for a more detailed discussion on the topic of AIDS family films.

16. Pagination for the English translation is from the George Braziller edition, *The Compassion Protocol.* Pagination from the French text is from the original Gallimard "Collection Blanche" edition. I will henceforth use the abbreviation *PC.*

17. The heterosexual subject is always masculine since its existence depends on the objectification of the feminine.

18. Guibert, "J'ai l'impression de survivre," 106. For more detailed information on what happened with the broadcast of the film, see Jean-Pierre Boulé, "The Postponing of *La pudeur ou l'impudeur.*" For more on the film itself see Ross Chambers, "The Suicide Experiment" and *Facing It.*

19. See Philippe Mangeot, "Subversion, transgression, follisation."

20. See in particular Laura Mulvey, "Visual Pleasure and Narrative Cinema," and Teresa de Lauretis, *Alice Doesn't*.

21. The expression "writing of disaster" is borrowed from Maurice Blanchot's *L'écriture du désastre*.

22. Derrida, *Dissemination*, 149.

23. Braudeau, "Ecrire contre la montre," 30.

24. See Didier Eribon, *Michel Foucault*, 336–37.

25. Ross Chambers, "Histoire d'Oeuf," 67.

26. Douglas Crimp, "Right On, Girlfriend!" 13.

27. Patricia Meyer Spacks, *Gossip*, 262.

28. I use the phrase "somewhat openly gay" to refer to the specifically French conditions of coming out, and, in the case of celebrities, the reluctance on the part of the media to make a public event out of a person's explicit mentions of his or her homosexuality. Let's just say that Thierry Le Luron was sufficiently open about his sexuality to allow rumors about his illness to spread quickly.

29. "I have read and heard all sorts of often sinister rumors, always coming from reliable yet sour sources [the French contains an untranslatable pun] . . . and spread by two thousand high society Parisian assholes, a scene made up of pathetic faggots who revel in muck" ["J'ai lu et entendu les bruits les plus divers, les plus sinistres aussi, toujours évidemment de source sûre, c'est-à-dire aigre . . . que colportent les deux mille cons du Tout-Paris, un milieu de tapettes insignifiantes qui ne se complaisent que dans la fiente"]. Quoted from *Le point*, 17 Nov. 1986, in Jérôme Strazzula, *Le sida 1981–1985*, 91. Strazzula's book is my main source of factual information concerning the Le Luron episode, but I've also relied on my own experience of these events.

30. Strazzula, *Le sida 1981–1985*, 94.

31. See in particular Douglas Crimp's criticism of Nicholas Nixon's photographs of PWAs in "Portraits of People with AIDS."

32. Jacques Almira, "D'un roman l'autre," 199. Interestingly enough, the remark is also framed in terms of national identity, or Frenchness. This suggests that Guibert must be a traitor not only to his friends but also to his country. Almira implies that Guibert's way of talking about AIDS is essentially un-French, and he unwittingly recognizes that the novels did in fact disrupt a certain high-cultural pattern of writing about sexuality and illness. While canonical, then, Guibert is also disrupting the canon.

Conclusion: French Universalism and the Question of Community

1. Quoted by Crimp, "Right On, Girlfriend!" 4. Vito Russo has since died.

2. Duplay, "Action = Vie," 56.

3. See "Tolérance," and Alain Royer and Christian Legrand, "Le drapeau gay interdit?"

4. See among others Rogers Brubaker, *Citizenship and Nationhood in France and Germany*, and Alec G. Hargreaves, *Immigration, "Race" and Ethnicity in Contemporary France*.

5. See Alain Touraine, "Faux et vrais problèmes" and *Pourrons-nous vivre ensemble?*

6. See for instance Alain Finkielkraut, "Le communautarisme est hideux."

7. The reception of Martel's book in France was not unlike that of Randy Shilts's *And the Band Played On* in the United States. It too was praised as a rigorous piece of investigative journalism conducted by a gay man, while its many homophobic clichés were given enhanced credence thanks to the gayness of their author.

8. See Etienne Balibar and Immanuel Wallerstein, *Race, nation, classe;* Maxim Silverman, *Deconstructing the Nation;* Michel Wieviorka, "Culture, société et démocratie."

9. See Brubaker, who shows the complexity of that opposition.

10. The purpose of this oversimplification is to make deportations more culturally acceptable in a country that still likes to describe itself as *terre d'asile* and *la patrie des droits de l'homme.*

11. On the social exclusion of categories defined as outside reason, see Touraine, "Faux et vrais problèmes," 297. Although he is referring to women, the observation is also valid for the figure of the "homosexual" as constructed by late nineteenth-century medical discourse. See chapter 1 of this book.

12. At this point I should make it clear that what I mean by "France" is the narrative of France, that is, the republican model described earlier, and not some essentialized cultural characteristic. In that sense it does include many gay men as well.

13. See Foucault, *The History of Sexuality,* vol. 1, 43 (*La volonté de savoir,* 59). For a discussion of the inherent instability of the figure of the homosexual as constructed by medical discourses in the second half of the nineteenth century, see chapter 1 of this book.

14. See Frank Arnal, *Résister ou disparaître?;* Yves Roussel, "Le mouvement homosexuel français face aux stratégies identitaires"; and Frédéric Martel, *Le rose et le noir.*

15. On this aspect of life in the Marais, see in particular Guillaume Dustan's brilliantly ironic novels *Dans ma chambre, Je sors ce soir, Plus fort que moi,* and *Nicolas Pages.* Dustan's work, in fact, can be read as a commentary on the traditional role of the French novel in performing communities.

16. This line of thinking was inspired by Todd Reeser's work on how, in Renaissance culture, ideal masculinity was defined as moderate against not one but two immoderate others, namely femininity and sodomy, thus allowing the emerging middle class to construct itself as moderate, too, and therefore better suited for political power. See "Framing Masculinity."

17. On the issue of conceiving and organizing IV drug users as a community, see Eric Lamien, "La communauté des drogués?"

18. In her weekly column in *Le nouvel observateur,* journalist Françoise Giroud, who presents herself as supportive of the rights of gays and lesbians, called François a "caricatural homosexual" ["caricature de l'homosexuel"] and wrote: "But it's . . . as if one had thrown a bucket of ice water on the very people who were asked to contribute, and who, by the the way . . . recanted. . . . Simply put, each time they [homosexuals] defy those who are irritated by their peculiar lifestyle, they make their own cause take one step back" ["Mais c'est . . . comme si l'on avait ouvert une douche froide sur ceux-là même dont on

sollicitait l'obole et qui, d'ailleurs . . . se sont rétractés. . . . Simplement, chaque fois qu'ils provoquent ceux que leurs moeurs particulières hérissent, ils font faire à leur cause un pas en arrière"] ("Les limites de la provoc"). Mireille Rosello called Martet's gesture "incredibly clumsy and incredibly understandable" ["incroyablement maladroit et incroyablement compréhensible"] ("Contamination et pureté," 11). She's probably right. For the next production of the *Sidaction,* in 1998, AIDS organizations were not allowed so much air time. It was also a disappointing failure in terms of funds collected. For more on the *Sidaction,* see Alain Ménil, *Sain[t]s et saufs.*

19. On the concepts of culture in French far-right politics, and particularly in Barrès, see David Carroll, *French Literary Fascism,* especially chapter 1, "The Use and Abuse of Culture."

20. In an interesting feminist reversal of that metaphor, Christine Delphy portrays the Republic as a pimp, to show how universal integration is an act of violence against the individual citizens it claims to protect. She writes:

> The torturer was the healer, and the healer was the bleeder: here's the truth about liberalism, whether hiding under the cloak of republican universalism (aka humanitarian liberalism, aka liberal humanitarianism), or under the more familiar appearance of the abusive parent, the possessive lover, the harasser, the violent husband. The pimp is the archetype of this figure—hitting and comforting, comforting and hitting.

> [Le bourreau était le soigneur, le soigneur était le saigneur: voilà la vérité du libéralisme, qu'il se cache sous les dehors de l'universalisme républicain (*alias* libéralisme humanitaire, *alias* humanitarisme libéral), ou sous ceux plus connus du parent abusif, de l'amoureux possessif, du harceleur, du mari violent. Le souteneur est l'archétype de cette figure. Qui cogne et qui console. Qui console et qui cogne]. ("L'humanitarisme républicain contre les mouvements homos," 22)

BIBLIOGRAPHY

ACT UP-Paris. *Le sida: Combien de divisions?* Paris: Dagorno, 1994.

A Daughter's Diary. Dir. Nicole Betancourt. JDD Films, 1995.

Aggelton, Peter, and Hilary Homans, eds. *Social Aspects of AIDS.* London: Falmer Press, 1988.

Alcorn, Keith. "Illness, Metaphor and AIDS." In Aggelton and Homans, eds., *Social Aspects of AIDS,* 65–82.

Almira, Jacques. "D'un roman l'autre." Rev. of *A l'ami qui ne m'a pas sauvé la vie* by Hervé Guibert. *La revue des deux mondes,* April 1990, 196–201.

An Early Frost. Dir. John Erman. NBC, 1985.

Apter, Emily. "Fantom Images: Hervé Guibert and the Writing of 'sida' in France." In Murphy and Poirier, eds., *Writing AIDS,* 83–97.

Aristotle, *The Art of Rhetoric.* London: Penguin Books, 1991.

Armengaud, André. *La population française au XIXème siècle.* Paris: PUF, 1971.

Arnal, Frank. *Résister ou disparaître? Les homosexuels face au sida: la prévention de 1982 à 1992.* Paris: L'Harmattan, 1993.

Baguley, David. "Le récit de guerre: narration et focalisation dans *La débâcle.*" *Littérature* 50 (May 1983): 77–90.

Balibar, Etienne, and Immanuel Wallerstein. *Race, nation, classe: les identités ambiguës.* Paris: La Découverte, 1988.

Barbedette, Gilles. *Mémoires d'un jeune homme devenu vieux.* Paris: Gallimard, 1993.

Barthes, Roland. *Le degré zéro de l'écriture.* Paris: Seuil, 1953.

Barthes, Roland. *Littérature et réalité.* Paris: Seuil, 1982.

Bataille, Georges. *Literature and Evil.* Trans. Alastair Hamilton. London: Calder & Boyars Ltd, 1973. Trans. of *La littérature et le mal.* Paris: Gallimard, 1957.

Bataille, Georges. *Oeuvres complètes.* 12 vols. Paris: Gallimard, 1970–1988.

Baverel, Philippe. "Le drapeau gay flotte rue Sainte-Croix-de-la-Bretonnerie." *Le monde,* 22 June 1996, 11.

Beer, Gillian. "Plot and the Analogy with Science in Later Nineteenth Century Novelists." *Comparative Criticism: A Yearbook* 2 (1980): 131–49.

Beizer, Janet. "The Body in Question: Anatomy, Textuality, and Fetishism in Zola." *L'esprit créateur* 29, no. 1 (spring 1989): 50–60.

Beizer, Janet. *Ventriloquized Bodies: Narratives of Hysteria in Nineteenth-Century France.* Ithaca, N.Y.: Cornell University Press, 1994.

Bellour, Raymond. "Trompe-la-mort." Rev. of *A l'ami qui ne m'apas sauvé la vie* by Hervé Guibert. *Le magazine littéraire* 276, April 1990, 54–56.

Bergen, Véronique. *Jean Genet: entre mythe et réalité.* Bruxelles: De Boeck-Wesmael, 1993.

Bernstein, Michele. "Celui qui 'parle par sa bouche.'" Rev. of *Les gangsters* and *Mauve le vierge* by Hervé Guibert. *Libération,* 20 Oct. 1988, xii.

Bernstein, Michele. "Hervé Guibert: Une écriture charismatique." Rev. of *Cytomégalovirus* and *L'homme au chapeau rouge* by Hervé Guibert. *Libération,* 30 Jan. 1992, 23.

Bersani, Leo. *Homos.* Cambridge, Mass.: Harvard University Press, 1995.

Bersani, Leo. "Is the Rectum a Grave?" In Crimp, ed., *AIDS: Cultural Analysis, Cultural Activism,* 197–222.

Bianciotti, Hector. "La mort d'Hervé Guibert: jusqu'au bout de la nuit." *Le monde,* 29–30 Dec. 1991, 1+.

Bickel, Gisèle A. Child. *Jean Genet: criminalité et transcendance.* Saratoga: Anma Libri, 1987.

Blanchot, Maurice. *L'écriture du désastre.* Paris: Gallimard, 1980.

Boffin, Tessa, and Sunil Gupta, eds. *Ecstatic Antibodies: Resisting the AIDS Mythology.* London: Rivers Oram Press, 1990.

Bonnefoy, Claude. *Jean Genet.* Paris: Editions Universitaires, 1965.

Borie, Jean. *Mythologies de l'hérédité au XIXème siècle.* Paris: Galilée, 1981.

Boulé, Jean-Pierre. "Hervé Guibert à la télévision: vérité et séduction." *Nottingham French Studies* 34, no. 1 (spring 1995): 112–20.

Boulé, Jean-Pierre. *Hervé Guibert: A l'ami qui ne m'a pas sauvé la vie and Other Writings.* Glasgow: University of Glasgow French and German Publications, 1995.

Boulé, Jean-Pierre. "Introduction." In *Hervé Guibert,* ed. Jean-Pierre Boulé. Special issue. *Nottingham French Studies* 34, no. 1 (spring 1995): 1–4.

Boulé, Jean-Pierre. "The Postponing of *La pudeur ou l'impudeur:* Modesty or Hypocrisy on the Part of French Television?" *French Cultural Studies* 3 (Oct. 1992): 299–305.

Bourdieu, Pierre. *The Rules of Art: Genesis and Structure of the Literary Field.* Trans. Susan Emanuel. Stanford: Stanford University Press, 1995. Trans. of *Les règles de l'art: genèse et structure du champ littéraire.* Paris: Plon, 1992.

Braudeau, Michel. "Ecrire contre la montre." *Le monde,* 2 March 1990, 30.

Bristow, Joseph, ed. "Lesbian and Gay Cultures: Theories and Texts." Special issue. *Textual Practice* 4, no. 2 (summer 1990).

Brooks, Peter, and Joseph Halpern, eds. *Genet, a Collection of Critical Essays.* Englewood Cliffs, N.J.: Prentice Hall, 1979.

Brown, Frederick. *Zola: A Life.* New York: Farrar, Straus & Giroux, 1995.

Brubaker, Rogers. *Citizenship and Nationhood in France and Germany.* Cambridge, Mass.: Harvard University Press, 1992.

Butler, Judith. *Bodies That Matter: On the Discursive Limits of Sex.* New York: Routledge, 1993.

Butler, Judith. *Gender Trouble: Feminism and the Subversion of Identity.* New York: Routledge, 1990.

Butters, Ronald R., John M. Clum, and Michael Moon, eds. *Displacing Homophobia: Gay Male Perspectives in Literature and Culture*. Durham, N. C.: Duke University Press, 1989. Orig. publ. in *South Atlantic Quarterly* 88, no. 1 (winter 1989).

Canguilhem, Georges. *The Normal and the Pathological*. Trans. Carolyn R. Fawcett. New York: Zone Books, 1989. Trans. of *Le normal et le pathologique*. Paris: PUF, 1966.

Carlson, Eric T. "Medicine and Degeneration: Theory and Praxis." In Chamberlin and Gilman, eds., *Degeneration*, 121–44.

Caron, David. "Intrusions: The Family in AIDS Films." *L'esprit créateur* 38, no. 3 (fall 1998): 62–72.

Caron, David. "Liberté, Egalité, Séropositivité: AIDS, the French Republic, and the Question of Community." *French Cultural Studies* 9, no. 3 (Oct. 1998): 281–93.

Caron, David. "Playing Doctors: Refiguring the Doctor-Patient Relationship in Hervé Guibert's AIDS Novels." *Literature and Medicine* 14, no. 2 (fall 1995): 237–49.

Carroll, David. *French Literary Fascism: Nationalism, Anti-Semitism, and the Ideology of Culture*. Princeton, N.J.: Princeton University Press, 1995.

Carter, Erica, and Simon Watney, eds. *Taking Liberties: AIDS and Cultural Politics*. London: Serpent's Tail, 1989.

Chamberlin, J. Edward. "Images of Degeneration: Turnings and Transformations." In Chamberlin and Gilman, eds., *Degeneration*, 263–89.

Chamberlin, J. Edward, and Sander L. Gilman, eds. *Degeneration: The Dark Side of Progress*. New York: Columbia University Press, 1985.

Chamberlin, J. Edward, and Sander L. Gilman. "Introduction." In Chamberlin and Gilman, eds., *Degeneration*, ix–xiv.

Chambers, Ross. *Facing It: AIDS Diaries and the Death of the Author*. Ann Arbor: Univeristy of Michigan Press, 1999.

Chambers, Ross. "Gossip and the Novel: Knowing Narrative and Narrative Knowing in Balzac, Mme de Lafayette and Proust." *Australian Journal of French Studies* 23, no. 2 (1986): 212–33.

Chambers, Ross. "Histoire d'Oeuf: Secrets and Secrecy in a La Fontaine Fable." *SubStance* 32 (1981): 65–74.

Chambers, Ross. *Room for Maneuver: Reading (the) Oppositional (in) Narrative*. Chicago: University of Chicago Press, 1991.

Chambers, Ross. "The Suicide Experiment: Hervé Guibert's AIDS Video, *La pudeur ou l'impudeur*." *L'esprit créateur* 37, no. 3 (fall 1997): 72–82.

Citti, Pierre. *Contre la décadence: histoire de l'imagination française dans le roman, 1890–1914*. Paris: PUF, 1987.

Coe, Richard N. *The Vision of Jean Genet*. London: Peter Owen, 1968.

Cohen, Ed. "Legislating the Norm: From Sodomy to Gross Indecency." In Butters, Clum, and Moon, eds., *Displacing Homophobia*, 169–205.

Colatrella, Carol. "Representing Liberty: Revolution, Sexuality, and Science in Michelet's Histories and Zola's Fictions." *Nineteenth-Century French Studies* 20, nos. 1–2 (fall–winter 1991–1992): 27–43.

Collard, Cyril. *Les nuits fauves*. Paris: Flammarion, 1989.

"Communautarisme ou républicanisme?" *Ex aequo* 8 (June 1997): 38–49.

Compagnon, Antoine. "Zola dans la décadence." *Les cahiers naturalistes* 67 (1993): 11–22.

Copi. *Une visite inopportune*. Paris: Bourgois, 1988.

Copley, Antony. *Sexual Moralities in France, 1780–1980: Ideas on the Family, Divorce, and Homosexuality*. London: Routledge, 1989.

Craft, Christopher. "'Kiss me with those red lips': Gender and Inversion in Bram Stoker's *Dracula*." In *Speaking of Gender*, ed. Elaine Showalter, 216–42. New York: Routledge, 1989.

Crary, Jonathan, and Sandford Kwinter, eds. *Incorporations*. *Zone* 6. Cambridge, Mass.: MIT Press, 1992.

Crimp, Douglas, ed. *AIDS: Cultural Analysis, Cultural Activism*. Cambridge, Mass.: MIT Press, 1988. Orig. publ. in *October* 43 (1987).

Crimp, Douglas. "AIDS: Cultural Analysis, Cultural Activism." In Crimp, ed., *AIDS: Cultural Analysis, Cultural Activism*, 3–16.

Crimp, Douglas. "How to Have Promiscuity in an Epidemic." In Crimp, ed., *AIDS: Cultural Analysis, Cultural Activism*, 237–71.

Crimp, Douglas. "Mourning and Militancy." *October* 51 (winter 1989): 3–18.

Crimp, Douglas. "Portraits of People with AIDS." In Stanton, ed., *Discourses of Sexuality*, 362–88.

Crimp, Douglas. "Right On, Girlfriend!" *Social Text* 33 (1992): 2–18.

Crimp, Douglas, with Adam Rolston. *AIDS Demo Graphics*. Seattle: Bay Press, 1990.

Deleuze, Gilles. *Logique du sens*. Paris: Minuit, 1969.

Deleuze, Gilles, and Félix Guattari. *L'anti-Oedipe: capitalisme et schizophrénie*. Paris: Minuit, 1972.

Deleuze, Gilles, and Félix Guattari. *Mille plateaux: capitalisme et schizophrénie*. Paris: Minuit, 1980.

Delphy, Christine. "L'humanitarisme républicain contre les mouvements homos." *Politique, la revue* 5 (July–Sept. 1997): 19–22.

Delvaux, Martine. "Des corps et des frontières: les lieux du sida." *L'esprit créateur* 37, no. 3 (fall 1997): 83–93.

Derrida, Jacques. *Dissemination*. Trans. Barbara Johnson. Chicago: University of Chicago Press, 1981. Trans. of *La dissémination*. Paris: Seuil, 1972.

Derrida, Jacques. *Glas*. Trans. John P. Leavy Jr. and Richard Rand. Lincoln: University of Nebraska Press, 1986. Trans. of *Glas*. Paris: Galilée, 1974.

Descotes, Maurice. "Le personnage de Napoléon III dans *Les Rougon-Macquart*." *Archives des lettres modernes* 6 (1970): 1–79.

Deslhiat, Claude. "L'aveuglement des années 1982–1985 et ses causes." In *Sida, sexe et société*. Special issue. *Regards sur l'actualité* 194–195 (Sept.–Nov. 1993): 25–55.

Dichy, Albert, and Pascal Fouché. *Jean Genet: essai de chronologie, 1910–1944*. Paris: Bibliothèque de littérature contemporaine de l'Université Paris VII, 1988.

Dollimore, Jonathan. *Sexual Dissidence: Augustine to Wilde, Freud to Foucault.* Oxford: Clarendon Press, 1991.

Douglas, Mary. *Purity and Danger.* New York: Praeger, 1970.

Drescher, Seymour, David Sabean, and Allan Sharlin, eds. *Political Symbolism in Modern Europe.* New Brunswick, N.J.: Transaction, 1982.

Dreuilhe, Alain Emmanuel. *Corps à corps: journal de sida.* Paris: Gallimard, 1987.

Duncan, Derek. "Gestes autobiographiques: le sida et les formes d'expressions artistiques du moi." *Nottingham French Studies* 34, no. 1 (spring 1995): 100–111.

Duplay, Mathieu. "Action = Vie." In "Sida: le combat," 56.

Durham, Scott. "Editor's Preface: In the Language of the Enemy." *Yale French Studies* 91 (1997): 1–6.

Durham, Scott, ed. "Genet: In the Language of the Enemy." Special issue. *Yale French Studies* 91 (1997).

Dustan, Guillaume. *Dans ma chambre.* Paris: P.O.L, 1996.

Dustan, Guillaume. *Je sors ce soir.* Paris: P.O.L, 1997.

Dustan, Guillaume. *Nicolas Pages.* Paris: Balland, 1999.

Dustan, Guillaume. *Plus fort que moi.* Paris: P.O.L, 1998.

Duve, Pascal de. *Cargo Vie.* Paris: Lattès, 1993.

Dyer, Richard. "Children of the Night: Vampirism as Homosexuality, Homosexuality as Vampirism." In Radstone, ed., *Sweet Dreams,* 47–72.

Edelman, Lee. "The Mirror and the Tank: 'AIDS,' Subjectivity, and the Rhetoric of Activism." In Murphy and Poirier, eds., *Writing AIDS,* 9–38.

Edelman, Lee. "The Plague of Discourse: Politics, Literary Theory, and AIDS." In Butters, Clum, and Moon, eds., *Displacing Homophobia,* 289–305.

Edelman, Lee. "Seeing Things: Representations, the Scene of Surveillance, and the Spectacle of Gay Male Sex." In Fuss, ed., *Inside/Out,* 93–116.

Eknoyan, Garabed, and Byron A. Eknoyan. "Medicine and the Case of Emile Zola." In *The Body and the Text: Comparative Essays in Literature and Medicine,* ed. Wendell Aycock, 103–14. Lubbock: Texas Tech University Press, 1990.

Ekotto, Frieda. *L'écriture carcérale et le discours juridique chez Jean Genet et Roger Knobelspiess.* Paris: L'Harmattan, 2001.

Eribon, Didier. *Michel Foucault.* Paris: Flammarion, 1989.

Eribon, Didier. *Michel Foucault et ses contemporains.* Paris: Fayard, 1994.

Erni, John Nguyet. *Unstable Frontiers: Technomedicine and the Cultural Politics of "Curing" AIDS.* Minneapolis: University of Minnesota Press, 1994.

Feldman, Douglas A., ed. *Culture and AIDS.* New York: Praeger, 1990.

Fernandez, Dominique. *La gloire du paria.* Paris: Grasset, 1987.

Fernandez, Dominique. "La liberté, tombeau de l'inspiration." *Le Nouvel observateur,* 18–24 Feb. 1993, 10–11.

Fernandez, Dominique. *Le rapt de Ganymède.* Paris: Grasset, 1989.

Finkielkraut, Alain. "Le communautarisme est hideux." Interview with Olivier Razemon. *Ex aequo* 8 (June 1997): 44.

Foucault, Michel. *Birth of the Clinic: An Archeology of Medical Perception.* Trans. A. M. Sheridan Smith. New York: Pantheon Books, 1973. Trans. of *Naissance de la clinique.* Paris: PUF, 1963.

Foucault, Michel. *The History of Sexuality*, vol. 1: *An Introduction.* Trans. Robert Hurley. New York: Vintage Books, 1980. Trans. of *La volonté de savoir.* Paris: Gallimard, 1976. Vol. 1 of *Histoire de la sexualité.* 3 vols. 1976–1984.

Foucault, Michel. *Madness and Civilization: A History of Insanity in the Age of Reason.* Trans. Richard Howard. New York: Pantheon, 1965. Trans. of *Folie et déraison: histoire de la folie à l'âge classique.* Paris: Plon, 1961.

Foucault, Michel. "What Is an Author?" In *Textual Strategies: Perspective in Post-Structuralist Criticism*, ed. Josué V. Harari, 141–60. Ithaca, N.Y.: Cornell University Press, 1979.

Fuss, Diana, ed. *Inside/Out: Lesbian Theories, Gay Theories.* New York: Routledge, 1991.

Gaudemar, Antoine de. "Hervé Guibert, la mort propagande." *Libération*, 28–29 Dec. 1991, 25–27.

Gehler, Monique. "La tragédie homosexuelle." *L'évènement du jeudi*, 3 Dec. 1992, 70–82.

Genet, Jean. *Journal du voleur, Querelle de Brest, Pompes funèbres.* Paris: Gallimard (Biblos), 1993.

Genet, Jean. *Oeuvres complètes.* 6 vols. Paris: Gallimard, 1951–1991.

Genet, Jean. *Our Lady of the Flowers.* Trans. Bernard Frechtman. New York: Grove Press, 1963. Trans. of *Notre-Dame-des-fleurs.* Lyon: L'Arbalète, 1943.

Genet, Jean. *Querelle.* Trans. Anselm Hollo. New York, Grove Press, 1974. Trans. of *Querelle de Brest.* Paris: Gallimard, 1953.

Genet, Jean. *The Thief's Journal.* Trans. Bernard Frechtman. New York: Grove Press, 1964. Trans. of *Journal du voleur.* Paris: Gallimard, 1949.

Gever, Martha. "Pictures of Sickness: Stuart Marshall's *Bright Eyes.*" In Crimp, ed., *AIDS: Cultural Analysis, Cultural Activism*, 109–26.

Gide, André. *Paludes.* Paris: Gallimard, 1926.

Gide, André. *Prétextes.* Paris: Mercure de France, 1947.

Gilman, Sander L. "AIDS and Syphilis: The Iconography of Disease." In Crimp, ed., *AIDS: Cultural Analysis, Cultural Activism*, 87–108.

Gilman, Sander L. *Difference and Pathology: Stereotypes of Sexuality, Race, and Madness.* Ithaca, N.Y.: Cornell University Press, 1985.

Gilman, Sander L. *Disease and Representation: Images of Illness from Madness to AIDS.* Ithaca, N.Y.: Cornell University Press, 1988.

Gilman, Sander L. *The Jew's Body.* New York: Routledge, 1991.

Gilman, Sander L. "Sexology, Psychoanalysis, and Degeneration: From a Theory of Race to a Race to Theory." In Chamberlin and Gilman, eds., *Degeneration*, 72–96.

Gilman, Sander L., and Steven T. Katz, eds. *Anti-Semitism in Times of Crisis.* New York: New York University Press, 1991.

Gilman, Stuart C. "Political Theory and Degeneration: From Left to Right, from Up to Down." In Chamberlin and Gilman, eds., *Degeneration*, 165–98.

Giroud, Françoise. "Les limites de la provoc," *Le nouvel observateur*, 13–19 June 1996, 55.

Glissant, Edouard. *Poétique de la Relation*. Paris: Gallimard, 1990.

Greenberg, David F. *The Construction of Homosexuality*. Chicago: Chicago University Press, 1988.

Grover, Jan Zita. "Constitutional Symptoms." In Carter and Watney, eds., *Taking Liberties*, 147–59.

Grover, Jan Zita. "Visible Lesions: Images of People with AIDS." *Afterimage* 17, no. 1 (1989): 10–16.

Guibert, Hervé. "Les aveux permanents d'Hervé Guibert." Interview with Antoine de Gaudemar. *Libération*, 20 Oct. 1988, xii.

Guibert, Hervé. *The Compassion Protocol*. Trans. James Kirkup. New York: George Braziller, 1994. Trans. of *Le protocole compassionnel*. Paris: Gallimard, 1991.

Guibert, Hervé. *Cytomégalovirus*. Paris: Seuil, 1992.

Guibert, Hervé. "Foucault a été mon maître, je devais écrire sa mort . . . " Interview with Philippe Lançon. *L'événement du jeudi*, 1–7 March 1990, 82–85.

Guibert, Hervé. "Hervé Guibert et son double." Interview with Didier Eribon. *Le nouvel observateur*, 18–24 July 1991, 87–89.

Guibert, Hervé. *L'homme au chapeau rouge*. Paris: Gallimard, 1992.

Guibert, Hervé. "J'ai l'impression de survivre." Interview. *L'événement du jeudi*, 26 Sept.–2 Oct. 1991, 104–6.

Guibert, Hervé. *Mes parents*. Paris: Gallimard, 1986.

Guibert, Hervé. *To the Friend Who Did Not Save My Life*. Trans. Linda Coverdale. New York: Atheneum, 1994. Trans. of *A l'ami qui ne m'a pas sauvé la vie*. Paris: Gallimard, 1990.

Guibert, Hervé. "La vie sida." Interview with Antoine de Gaudemar. *Libération*, 1 March 1990, 19–21.

Halperin, David M. *Saint Foucault: Towards a Gay Hagiography*. New York: Oxford University Press, 1995.

Hanson, Ellis. "Undead." In Fuss, ed., *Inside/Out*, 324–40.

Haraway, Donna Jeanne. *Crystals, Fabrics, and Fields: Metaphors of Organicism in Twentieth-Century Developmental Biology*. New Haven: Yale University Press, 1976.

Hargreaves, Alec G. *Immigration, "Race" and Ethnicity in Contemporary France*. London: Routledge, 1995.

Hauptman, Robert. *The Pathological Vision: Jean Genet, Louis-Ferdinand Céline, and Tennessee Williams*. New York: P. Lang, 1984.

Hill, Leslie. "Ecrire—la maladie." *Nottingham French Studies* 34, no. 1 (spring 1995): 89–99.

Hillenaar, Henk. "Hervé Guibert (1955–1991)." In *Jeunes auteurs de Minuit*, ed. Michèle Ammouche-Kremers and Henk Hillenaar, 95–102. Amsterdam: Rodopi, 1994.

Hirsch, William. *Genius and Degeneration*. London: Heinemann, 1897.

Hocquenghem, Guy. *Eve*. Paris: Albin Michel, 1987.

Hocquenghem, Guy. *Homosexual Desire*. Trans. Daniella Dangoor. London: Allison & Busby, 1978. Trans. of *Le désir homosexuel*. Paris: Editions universitaires, 1972.

In the Gloaming. Dir. Christopher Reeve. HBO-NYC, 1997.

"In Time of Plague." Special Issue. *Social Research* 55 (1988).

It's My Party. Dir. Randal Kleiser. United Artists, 1996.

Jaccomard, Hélène. "La thanatologie chez Hervé Guibert." *Journal of European Studies* 25 (Sept. 1995): 283–302.

Kaempfer, Jean. *Emile Zola: d'un naturalisme pervers*. Paris: José Corti, 1989.

Katz, Jonathan Ned. *The Invention of Heterosexuality*. New York: Dutton, 1995.

Keller, Evelyn Fox. *Reflections on Gender and Science*. New Haven: Yale University Press, 1985.

King, Graham. *Garden of Zola*. New York: Barnes and Noble Books, 1978.

Krafft-Ebing, Richard von. *Psychopathia Sexualis*. Paris: Payot, 1969.

Kramer, Larry. *The Normal Heart*. New York: Plume, 1985.

Kristeva, Julia. *Powers of Horror: An Essay on Abjection*. Trans. Leon S. Roudiez. New York: Columbia University Press, 1982. Trans. of *Pouvoirs de l'horreur: essai sur l'abjection*. Paris: Seuil, 1980.

Kuhn, Thomas. *Structures of Scientific Revolutions*. 2nd ed. Chicago: University of Chicago Press, 1970.

Lamien, Eric. "La communauté des drogués?" *Ex aequo* 7 (May 1997): 12–13.

Lanteri-Laura, Georges. *Lecture des perversions: histoire de leur appropriation médicale*. Paris: Masson, 1979.

Lapp, John. "The Watcher Betrayed and the Fatal Woman: Some Recurring Patterns in Zola." *PMLA* 74 (1959): 276–84.

La pudeur et l'impudeur. Dir. Hervé Guibert TF1. 30 Jan. 1992.

Laqueur, Thomas. *Making Sex: Body and Gender from the Greeks to Freud*. Cambridge, Mass.: Harvard University Press, 1990.

Laroche, Hadrien. *Le dernier Genet: histoire des hommes infâmes*. Paris: Seuil, 1997.

Laupts, Dr. [Saint-Paul, Georges]. *L'homosexualité et les types homosexuels*. Paris: Vigot, 1910.

Lauretis, Teresa de. *Alice Doesn't: Feminism, Semiotics, Cinema*. Bloomington: Indiana University Press, 1984.

Leap, William L. "Language and AIDS." In Feldman, ed., *Culture and AIDS*, 137–58.

Le Bon, Gustave. *Psychologie des foules*. Paris: PUF, 1947.

Ledes, Richard C., and Martin G. Koloski. "AIDS and the Ninjas." *Copyright* 1 (1987): 133–45.

Lefort, Gérard. "C'est l'histoire de Garçon Maigre." Rev. of *La pudeur et l'impudeur* by Hervé Guibert. *Libération*, 30 Jan. 1992, 46.

Leglulic, H. *Notes et observations de médecine légale*. Paris, 1895.

Lethbridge, Robert. "Zola: Decadence and Autobiography in the Genesis of a Fictional Character." *Nottingham French Studies* 17, no. 1 (May 1978): 39–51.

LeVay, Simon. *The Sexual Brain*. Cambridge, Mass.: MIT Press, 1993.

Macey, David. *The Lives of Michel Foucault: A Biography*. New York: Pantheon, 1993.

McNally, Terence. *Love! Valour! Compassion!* New York: Plume, 1995.

Malinas, Y. *Zola et les hérédités imaginaires*. Paris: Expansion Scientifique Françaises, 1985.

Mangeot, Philippe. "Subversion, transgression, follisation." *Ex aequo* 29 (July–Sept. 1999): 47.

Marsan, Hugo. *La vie blessée: le sida, l'ère du soupçon.* Paris: Maren Sell, 1989.

Marshall, Stuart. "Picturing Deviancy." In Boffin and Gupta, eds., *Ecstatic Antibodies,* 19–36.

Martel, Frédéric. "Guibert, Koltès, Copi: littérature et sida." *Esprit* 206 (Nov. 1994): 65–73.

Martel, Frédéric. *Le rose et le noir: les homosexuels en France depuis 1968.* Paris: Seuil, 1996.

Mathiot, Pierre. "Le sida dans la stratégie et la rhétorique du Front national." In *Sida et politique: les premiers affrontements (1981–1987),* ed. Pierre Favre, 189–201. Paris: L'Harmattan, 1992.

Maupassant, Guy de. *Le Horla.* Paris: Albin Michel, 1962.

"Medicine, History and Society." Special issue. *Journal of Contemporary History* 20 (1985).

Mendès-Leite, Rommel, and Pierre-Olivier de Busscher. "La gestion d'une épidémie à long terme." In "Sida: le combat," 22–23.

Ménil, Alain. *Sain[t]s et saufs. Sida: une épidémie de l'interprétation.* Paris: Les Belles Lettres, 1997.

Meyer, Richard. "Rock Hudson's Body." In Fuss, ed., *Inside/Out,* 259–88.

Moraly, Jean-Bernard. *Jean Genet: la vie écrite.* Paris: Éditions de la Différence, 1988.

Morel, Bénédict Augustin. *Traité des dégénérescences physiques, intellectuelles et morales de l'espèce humaine.* Paris, 1857.

Moscovici, Claudia. "Androgyny and Morality in *Germinal*." *Dalhousie French Studies* 20 (spring–summer 1991): 27–38.

Mosse, George L. *Nationalism and Sexuality: Respectabilty and Abnormal Sexuality in Modern Europe.* New York: Howard Fertig, 1985.

Mulvey, Laura. "Visual Pleasure and Narrative Cinema." *Screen* 16 (Aug. 1975): 6–18.

Murphy, Timothy F., and Suzanne Poirier, eds. *Writing AIDS: Gay Literature, Language, and Analysis.* New York: Columbia University Press, 1993.

Navarre, Max. "Fighting the Victim Label." In Crimp, ed., *AIDS: Cultural Analysis, Cultural Activism,* 143–46.

Navarre, Max. "PWA Coalition Portfolio." In Crimp, ed., *AIDS: Cultural Analysis, Cultural Activism,* 147–68.

Nordau, Max. *Degeneration.* New York: D. Appleton, 1895.

Nunokawa, Jeff. "'All the Sad Young Men': AIDS and the Work of Mourning." In Fuss, ed., *Inside/Out,* 311–23.

Nye, Robert A. "The Bio-Medical Origins of Urban Sociology." *Journal of Contemporary History* 20 (1985): 659–75.

Nye, Robert A. *Crime, Madness, and Politics in Modern France: The Medical Concept of National Decline.* Princeton, N.J.: Princeton University Press, 1984.

Nye, Robert A. "Degeneration and the Medical Model of Cultural Crisis in the French Belle Epoque." In Drescher, Sabean, and Sharlin, eds., *Political Symbolism in Modern Europe,* 19–41.

Our Sons. Dir. John Erman. ABC, 1991.

Paris Is Burning. Dir. Jennie Livingston. Prestige, 1992.

Patton, Brian. "Cell Wars: Military Metaphors and the Crisis of Authority in the AIDS Epidemic." In *Fluid Exchanges: Artists and Critics in the AIDS Crisis,* ed. James Miller, 272–86. Toronto: University of Toronto Press, 1992.

Patton, Cindy. *Fatal Advice.* Durham, N.C.: Duke University Press, 1996.

Patton, Cindy. *Inventing AIDS.* New York: Routledge, 1990.

Petrey, Sandy. "Anna-Nana-Nana: identité sexuelle, écriture naturaliste, lectures lesbiennes." *Les cahiers naturalistes* 41, no. 69 (1995): 69–80.

Petrey, Sandy. "La république de *La débâcle.*" *Les cahiers naturalistes* 54 (1980): 87–95.

Philadelphia. Dir. Jonathan Demme. Tristar, 1993.

Pick, Daniel. *Faces of Degeneration: A European Disorder, c.1848–c.1918.* Cambridge: Cambridge University Press, 1989.

Pike, Burton. *The Image of the City in Modern Literature.* Princeton, N.J.: Princeton University Press, 1981.

Rabinbach, Anson. "The Body without Fatigue: A Nineteenth-Century Utopia." In Drescher, Sabean, and Sharlin, eds., *Political Symbolism in Modern Europe,* 42–62.

Rabinbach, Anson. "Neurasthenia and Modernity." In Crary and Kwinter, eds., *Incorporations,* 178–89.

Radstone, Susannah, ed. *Sweet Dreams: Sexuality, Gender and Popular Fiction.* London: Lawrence and Wishart, 1988.

Reeser, Todd. "Framing Masculinity: The Discourse of Moderation in Renaissance Culture." Diss. University of Michigan, 1997.

Renan, Ernest. "Qu'est-ce qu'une nation?" *Discours et conférences.* Paris: Calmann-Lévy, 1887: 277–310.

Ricardou, Jean. *Le nouveau roman: hier, aujourd'hui.* Paris: UGE, 1972.

Ricardou, Jean. *Problèmes du nouveau roman.* Paris: Seuil, 1967.

Rieusset-Lemarié, Isabelle. *Une fin de siècle épidémique.* Paris: Actes Sud, 1992.

Robinson, Christopher. *Scandal in the Ink: Male and Female Homosexuality in Twentieth-Century French Literature.* London: Cassell, 1995.

Rosello, Mireille. "Contamination et pureté: pour un protocole de cohabitation." *L'Esprit créateur* 37, no. 3 (fall 1997): 3–13.

Rosen, Karl. "Emile Zola and Homosexuality." *Excavatio: Emile Zola and Naturalism* 2 (fall 1993): 111–15.

Roussel, Yves. "Le mouvement homosexuel français face aux stratégies identitaires." *Les temps modernes* 582 (May–June 1995): 85–108.

Royer, Alain, and Christian Legrand. "Le drapeau gay interdit?" *Têtu* 4 (June 1996), 12.

Rufener, Helen Beatrice. *Biography of a War Novel: Zola's "La débâcle."* New York: King's Crown Press, 1946.

Russo, Vito. *The Celluloid Closet: Homosexuality in the Movies.* Rev. ed. New York: Harper and Row, 1987.

Rutherford, J., ed. *Identity: Community, Culture, Difference.* London: Lawrence and Wishart, 1990.

Said, Edward. *Orientalism*. New York: Pantheon, 1978.

Sarkonak, Ralph. "De la métastase au métatexte," *Texte* 15–16 (1994): 229–59.

Sarkonak, Ralph. "Traces and Shadows: Fragments of Hervé Guibert." In *Same Sex/ Different Text? Gay and Lesbian Writing in French*, ed. Brigitte Mahuzier, Karen McPherson, Charles A. Porter, and Ralph Sarkonak. Special issue. *Yale French Studies* 90 (1996): 172–202.

Sartre, Jean-Paul. *Saint Genet, Actor and Martyr*. Trans. Bernard Frechtman. New York: George Braziller, 1963. Trans. of *Saint Genet, comédien et martyr*. Paris: Gallimard, 1952.

Schehr, Lawrence R. *Alcibiades at the Door: Gay Discourses in French Literature*. Stanford: Stanford University Press, 1995.

Schor, Naomi. "Mother's Day: Zola's Women." In *Critical Essays on Emile Zola*, ed. David Baguley, 130–41. Boston: Hall, 1986.

Schor, Naomi. *Zola's Crowds*. Baltimore, Md.: Johns Hopkins University Press, 1978.

Sedgwick, Eve Kosofsky. *Between Men: English Literature and Male Homosocial Desire*. New York: Columbia, 1985.

Sedgwick, Eve Kosofsky. "Epidemics of the Will." In Crary and Kwinter, eds., *Incorporations*, 582–95.

Sedgwick, Eve Kosofsky. *Epistemology of the Closet*. Berkeley: University of California Press, 1990.

Sell, Roger D. "Literary Gossip, Literary Theory, Literary Pragmatics." In *Literature and the New Interdisciplinarity: Poetics, Linguistics, History*, ed. Roger D. Sell and Peter Verdonk, 221–41. Atlanta: Rodopi, 1994.

Sellier, Bernard. "De la difficulté de vivre." In "Sida: le combat," 52.

Serres, Michel. *Feux et signaux de brume: Zola*. Paris: Grasset, 1975.

Sheringham, Michael. "Narration and Experience in Genet's *Journal du voleur*." In *Studies in French Fiction*, ed. Robert Gibson, 289–306. London: Grant and Cutler, 1988.

Sherry, Michael S. "The Language of War in AIDS Discourse." In Murphy and Poirier, eds., *Writing AIDS*, 39–53.

Shilts, Randy. *And the Band Played On: Politics, People, and the AIDS Epidemic*. New York: St. Martin's Press, 1987.

"Sida: le combat." Special issue. *Les lettres françaises* 1393 (June 1993).

SIDA'venture: SIDA, éthique, discriminations. Paris: Syllepse, 1989.

Silverman, Maxim. *Deconstructing the Nation: Immigration, Racism and Citizenship in Modern France*. London: Routledge, 1992.

Smith, John H. "Abulia: Sexuality and Diseases of the Will in the Late Nineteenth Century." *Genders* 6 (fall 1989): 102–23.

Sontag, Susan. *Illness as Metaphor* and *AIDS and Its Metaphors*. New York: Doubleday, 1990.

Spacks, Patricia Meyer. *Gossip*. New York: Alfred A. Knopf, 1985.

Stanton, Domna C., ed. *Discourses of Sexuality: From Aristotle to AIDS*. Ann Arbor: University of Michigan Press, 1992.

Stanton, Domna C. "Recuperating Women and the Man Behind the Screen." In *Sexuality and Gender in Modern Europe: Institutions, Texts, Images,* ed. James Grantham Turner, 247–65. Cambridge: Cambridge University Press, 1993.

Strazzula, Jérôme. *Le sida 1981–1985: les débuts d'une pandémie.* Paris: La Documentation Française, 1993.

Taylor, Christopher C. "AIDS and the Pathogenesis of Metaphor." In Feldman, ed., *Culture and AIDS,* 55–65.

Thoinot, Léon. *Attentats aux moeurs et perversion du sens génital.* Paris, 1898.

"Tolérance." *L'hétéroriste* 13 (June 1996): 2.

Tort, Patrick. "Du fascisme sanitaire." In "Sida: le combat," 43–44.

Touraine, Alain. "Faux et vrais problèmes." In Wieviorka, ed., *Une société fragmentée?* 291–319.

Touraine, Alain. *Pourrons-nous vivre ensemble? Egaux et différents.* Paris: Fayard, 1997.

Treichler, Paula A. "AIDS, Gender, and Biomedical Discourse: Current Contests for Meaning." In *AIDS: The Burdens of History,* ed. Elizabeth Fee and Daniel M. Fox, 190–266. Berkeley: University of California Press, 1988.

Treichler, Paula A. "AIDS, Homophobia, and Biomedical Discourse: An Epidemic of Signification." In Crimp, ed., *AIDS: Cultural Analysis, Cultural Activism,* 31–70.

Troyat, Henri. *Zola.* Paris: Flammarion, 1992.

Ulrich, Claire. "Le Marais, quartier général du lobby homosexuel." *L'événement du jeudi,* 20–26 June 1996, 28–29.

Van Buuren, Marten. *"Les Rougon-Macquart" d'Emile Zola: de la métaphore au mythe.* Paris: José Corti, 1986.

Walker, Philip. *Zola.* London: Routledge & Kegan Paul, 1985.

Warner, Michael. "Fear of a Queer Planet." *Social Text* 29 (1991): 3–17.

Watney, Simon. "AIDS, 'Moral Panic' Theory and Homophobia." In Aggelton and Homans, eds., *Social Aspects of AIDS,* 52–64.

Watney, Simon. "Photography and AIDS." In *The Critical Image: Essays on Contemporary Photography,* ed. Carol Squiers, 173–92. Seattle: Bay Press, 1990.

Watney, Simon. *Policing Desire: Pornography, AIDS, and the Media.* Minneapolis: University of Minnesota Press, 1987.

Watney, Simon. "Representing AIDS." In Boffin and Gupta, eds., *Ecstatic Antibodies,* 165–92.

Watney, Simon. "The Spectacle of AIDS." In Crimp, ed., *AIDS: Cultural Analysis, Cultural Activism,* 71–86.

Watney, Simon. "The Subject of AIDS." *Copyright* 1 (fall 1987): 125–31.

Watney, Simon. "Taking Liberties: An Introduction." In Carter and Watney, eds., *Taking Liberties,* 11–57.

Weeks, Jeffrey. "AIDS, Altruism, and the New Right." In Carter and Watney, *Taking Liberties,* 127–32.

Weeks, Jeffrey. "Love in a Cold Climate." In Aggelton and Homans, eds., *Social Aspects of AIDS,* 10–19.

Weeks, Jeffrey. "Post-modern AIDS?" In Boffin and Gupta, eds., *Ecstatic Antibodies,* 133–41.

Wetsel, David. "The Best of Times, the Worst of Times: The Emerging Literature of AIDS in France." In *AIDS: The Literary Response,* ed. Emmanuel S. Nelson, 95–113. New York: Twayne, 1992.

Whipen, Deb. "Science Fictions: The Making of a Medical Model for AIDS." In *Facing AIDS,* 38–53. Special issue. *Radical America* 20, no. 6 (Nov.–Dec. 1988).

White, Edmund. *Genet: A Biography.* New York: Alfred A. Knopf, 1993.

White, Edmund. "Hervé Guibert: Sade in Jeans." In *The Burning Library: Essays,* ed. David Bergman, 355–66. New York: Alfred A. Knopf, 1994.

White, Edmund. "The Novelist Thief." *Brick* 47 (winter 1993): 3–4.

Wieviorka, Michel. "Culture, société et démocratie." In Wieviorka, ed., *Une société fragmentée?* 11–60.

Wieviorka, Michel, ed. *Une société fragmentée? Le multiculturalisme en débat.* Paris: La Découverte/Poche, 1997.

Williamson, Judith. "Every Virus Tells a Story: The Meanings of HIV and AIDS." In Carter and Watney, eds., *Taking Liberties,* 69–80.

Worth, Fabienne. "Le sacré et le sida: les représentations de la sexualité et leurs contradictions en France, 1971–1996." *Les temps modernes* (Feb. 1997): 75–113.

Zeldin, Théodore. "Les médecins français (1848–1945)." In *L'haleine des faubourgs: ville, habitat et santé au XIXe siècle,* ed. Lion Murard and Patrick Zylberman. Special issue. *Recherches* 29 (Dec. 1977): 223–44.

Zola, Emile. *L'atelier de Zola: Textes et Journaux 1865–1870.* Ed. Martin Kanes. Genève: Droz, 1963.

Zola, Emile. *Correspondance.* 10 vols. Ed. B. H. Bakker. Montréal: Les presses de l'Université de Montréal, 1977.

Zola, Emile. *The Debacle.* Trans. John Hands. Chester Springs, Penn.: Dufour Editions, 1969; London: Elek Books, 1968. Trans. of *La débâcle.* Paris: Fasquelle, 1892.

Zola, Emile. *The Downfall: A Story of the Horrors of War.* Trans. E. A. Vizetelly. London: Chattoo and Windus, 1914. Trans. of *La débâcle.* Paris: Fasquelle, 1892.

Zola, Emile. *Oeuvres complètes.* 15 vols. Ed. Henri Mitterand. Paris: Cercle du Livre Précieux, 1956–1970.

Zola, Emile. *Les Rougon-Macquart.* 5 vols. Paris: Gallimard, 1960–1967.

INDEX

Abjection, 71; anal sex and, 76–79; crime and, 74–76; definition of, 172 *n21*; maternal, 78; personification and representation of, 79–80; unicorn as counterpart of, 90–92

Abulia: described, 22; Maurice in *La débâcle,* 53–54; Napoleon III in *La débâcle,* 49

Activism: of ACT UP-Paris, 149; ACT UP's subversive activism, 129–30; gay identity and, 155; as opposite of passivity and narcissism, 132

ACT UP: subversive activism of, 129–30

ACT UP-Paris, 113, 155; activism of, 149; Guibert criticized by, 112; Martet's confrontation with Douste-Blazy, 158–60

Adjani, Isabelle, 118, 140, 142, 145. *See also* Marine

Aging and the diseased subject, 134–35

Aides, 113

AIDS: authors as authorities on, 147; as constructed in France, 3, 142–43; criticism in context of AIDS discourse, 9–10, 98; deportations of HIV positive persons, 158–59; disease metaphors and, 9–10; education campaigns, 178 *n41*; epidemiology of, 101–2, 154–55, 159–60; knowledge/power disrupted by, 9; as metaphor, 3–4, 102–3; in overseas territories (DOM-TOM), 157–58; representations, 96–97, 145–46; sufferer as construct, 105–11; xenophobia and, 176 *n24*. *See also* AIDS discourse; *Le sida*

AIDS and Its Metaphors, 102

AIDS discourse: basic narratives (virus, cure, and epidemic), 100–102; celebrities in, 107; constructions in terms of past epidemics, 99–100; as context for AIDS criti-

cism, 97–98; cultural history of, 96–111; fragmentation *vs.* wholeness in narratives, 136–37; health/illness dichotomy, 106; personal narrative *vs.* social or political, 114–19; sufferer as construct in, 105–11; vampires in, 107–8; virus as PWA, 108–9

A l'ami qui ne m'a pas sauvé la vie, 15–16; compatibility with cultural model, 118; fragmented structure of, 136–38; gossip and rumors in, 139–40; loss of identity as patient, 133; Marine in, 133–34, 145; Muzil in, 139–40, 144–45

Amputation metaphor, 42–43, 58, 60

Anti-Semitism: Jews as cultural Other, 14, 25–26, 35–37; in Zola's work, 168 *n5*

Anus: privatization of and social order, 77

Authority: and anonymity in scientific discourse, 146–47; of authors, 146–48; discourses of, 68–69; of Maurice as narrator in *La débâcle,* 59–61; medical authority and the AIDS sufferer, 105–6

Bachelot, Dr. François, 103–4

Barrès, Maurice, 14, 160

Bataille, Georges: on Genet, 93, 172 *n21*

Begging as ritual, 67

Benkert, Karoly Maria, 23

Bernard, Claude, 27–29

Biomedical discourse. *See* Medical discourses

Birth of the Clinic, 8

Body: beauty of, 122–23; *Bodies That Matter,* 73; constructions of sex and gender, 7; image and construction of PWA, 109–10; individual as body politic, 49, 72; leprosy and, 66; as metaphor, 7, 8–9, 66; nation state as, 8–9; physical identification of otherness, 8, 24, 106–11

Photography: and construction of PWA, 109–10; disruption of medical gaze, 127–29; used to mediate medical gaze, 123–24

Physical characteristics as signs in discourses of *dégénérescence*: in *La débâcle*, 32–33, 49–50; of leper or Other, 66; Napoleon III, 49–50; Other identified by, 8, 24, 106–11; of PWA, 106

Plague as metaphor, 99

Politics: Front National, 13, 15, 103–4; Le Pen, Jean-Marie, 13, 103, 176 *n26*; metaphor and ideology, 12–13; Right and Left, 12–13; "We are the Left" coalition, 160–61. *See also* Activism

Pompes funèbres, 84

Power and power relationships: AIDS sufferers and medical authority, 105–6; in Doctor/Patient, 131; gaze and, 49–50; heredity, 26; secrecy and, 140

Power/knowledge, 9, 30

Presymbolic moments, 82, 90–92

Procreation, 47, 170 *n23*; abjection of the maternal, 78; literature equated with, 42–44. *See also* Regeneration

Le protocole compassionnel, 15–16, 114, 118; contamination by reading, 138–39; fiberoptic exam scene, 123–24, 138

Psychopathia Sexualis, 23

Public/private dichotomy: subverted by gossip and rumors, 141

La pudeur ou l'impudeur, 114

PWA. *See* People with AIDS

Querelle de Brest, 87, 173 *n27*

Rainbow flag controversy, 150

Reading: as contagion, 138–39

Regeneration: in *La débâcle*, 31, 40

Religion: Christianity in *La débâcle*, 57; degeneration theorists and, 18; discourse of, 5; influence of Catholic Church, 158; saintliness in *Journal du voleur*, 92–93; *signes ostentoires* banned, 151

Republic: communities as antithetical to, 152–54; Others in Third Republic culture, 17; as pimp, 182 *n20*

Rimbaud, Arthur, 165–66 *n10*

Romanticism: Guibert as ideal artist, 112; tuberculosis and, 99; Zola and, 43–45, 58–59

Rumors, 70–71

Russo, Vito, 149

Saintliness: in *Journal du voleur*, 92–93

Saint-Paul, Georges, 47–48, 167 *n19*, 168 *n12*

Same/Other dichotomy: in biomedical discourse, 21–22; sexual inversion as challenge to, 26; sexual pathology and, 22–27

Sartre, Jean-Paul: on Genet, 81

Science: literature as, 27–29; metaphors of, 4–9; as objective/subjective, 5–6; paradigm shifts and, 6; science-gender system, 6–7

Science-gender system, 6–7

Scientific discourse: anonymity and authority in, 146–47

Serres, Michel: on *La débâcle*, 38–39

Sex: AIDS education campaigns, 178 *n41*; anal sex and abjection in *Journal du voleur*, 76–79; constructions of sex and gender, 7, 42, 93; female sexuality, 166 *n11*; reading equated with, 138–39; sexual inversion as challenge to two-sex model, 26; sexual "pathology" and Same/Other dichotomy, 22–27

"Sexual orientation," 13; and the Republic, 152

Le sida (SIDA): vs. SIDA as term, 97–98; violence inherent in *sida* narratives, 124

Sidaction, 156–57; atypical PWA featured by, 156–57, 159, 177 *n36*; confrontation between Martet and Douste-Blazy, 158–60; neglect of overseas territories (DOM-TOM), 157–58; People with AIDS and, 157; use of celebrities, 156

Sol En Si (Solidarité Enfants Sida), 158

Sontag, Susan, 102; construction of AIDS, 99; *Illness as Metaphor*, 66; on victims, 110–11

Stereotypes: actor, 51; in construction of PWA, 109–10; gossips, 140, 143–44; of PWA, 114, 178 *n40*

Sterility, 19, 47

The Structure of Scientific Revolutions, 6